Diagnosis and Management
of Craniopharyngiomas

Andrea Lania • Anna Spada
Giovanni Lasio
Editors

Diagnosis and Management of Craniopharyngiomas

Key Current Topics

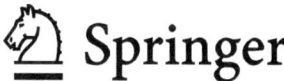 Springer

Editors
Andrea Lania
Department of Biomedical Sciences
Humanitas University
Rozzano
Italy

Giovanni Lasio
Neurosurgery Department
Istituto Clinico Humanitas
Rozzano (MI)
Italy

Anna Spada
DISCO Department Endocrinology
and Diabetology Unit
University of Milan IRCCS Fondazione
Policlinico Milano
Milan
Italy

ISBN 978-3-319-22296-7   ISBN 978-3-319-22297-4   (eBook)
DOI 10.1007/978-3-319-22297-4

Library of Congress Control Number: 2016937358

Printed on acid-free paper

This Springer imprint is published by Springer Nature
The registered company is Springer International Publishing AG Switzerland

Contents

Contributors

Luca Attuati, MD Department of Neurosurgery, Gamma Knife Unit, Humanitas Research Hospital, Rozzano, Italy

Michele Bailo Department of Neurosurgery, Vita-Salute University, San Raffaele Scientific Institute, Milan, Italy

Wenya Linda Bi Department of Neurosurgery, Brigham and Women's Hospital, Harvard Medical School, Boston, MA, USA

Gennaro D'Anna Department of Radiology, Humanitas Mater Domini, Castellanza, VA, Italy

Ian F. Dunn Department of Neurosurgery, Brigham and Women's Hospital, Harvard Medical School, Boston, MA, USA

Filippo Gagliardi Department of Neurosurgery, Vita-Salute University, San Raffaele Scientific Institute, Milan, Italy

Claudia Giavoli, MD Endocrinology and Diabetology Unit, Fondazione IRCCS Ospedale Maggiore IRCCS, Milan, Italy

Marco Grimaldi Neuroradiology Service, Humanitas Research Hospital, Rozzano, MI, Italy

Niki Karavitaki, MSc, PhD, FRCP Institute of Metabolism and Systems Research, College of Medical and Dental Sciences, University of Birmingham, Birmingham, UK

Centre for Endocrinology, Diabetes and Metabolism, Birmingham Health Partners, Birmingham, UK

Edward R. Laws Jr., MD Dana-Faber Cancer Institute, Boston, USA

Department of Neurosurgery, Brigham and Women's Hospital, Harvard Medical School, Boston, MA, USA

Marco Losa Department of Neurosurgery, Vita-Salute University, San Raffaele Scientific Institute, Milan, Italy

Juan Pedro Martinez-Barbera Birth Defects Research Centre, UCL Institute of Child Health, London, UK

Pietro Mortini Department of Neurosurgery and Radiosurgery, San Raffaele University Hospital, Milan, Italy

Department of Neurosurgery, Vita-Salute University, San Raffaele Scientific Institute, Milan, Italy

Breno Nery Department of Neurosurgery, Brigham and Women's Hospital, Harvard Medical School, Boston, MA, USA

Uberto Pagotto Division of Endocrinology, Department of Medical and Surgical Sciences, S. Orsola-Malpighi Hospital, University Alma Mater Studiorum of Bologna, Bologna, Italy

Division of Endocrinology, Department of Medical and Surgical Sciences, Centre for Applied Biomedical Research (C.R.B.A.), S. Orsola-Malpighi Hospital, University of Bologna, Bologna, Italy

Renato Pasquali Division of Endocrinology, Department of Medical and Surgical Science, Centre for Applied Biomedical Research (C.R.B.A.), S. Orsola-Malpighi Hospital, University of Bologna, Bologna, Italy

Alessandro Peri Department of Experimental and Clinical Biomedical Sciences "Mario Serio", Endocrine Unit, "Center for Research, Transfer and High Education on Chronic, Inflammatory, Degenerative and Neoplastic Disorders for the Development of Novel Therapies" (DENOThe), University of Florence, Florence, Italy

Piero Picozzi, MD Department of Neurosurgery, Gamma Knife Unit, Humanitas Research Hospital, Rozzano, Italy

Valentina Lo Preiato Division of Endocrinology, Department of Medical and Surgical Science, Centre for Applied Biomedical Research (C.R.B.A.), S. Orsola-Malpighi Hospital, University of Bologna, Bologna, Italy

Federico Roncaroli Departments of Medicine, Imperial College Healthcare Trust, London, UK

Division of Institute of Brain, Behaviour and Mental Health, The University of Manchester Institute of Child Health, University College of London, London, UK

Giuseppe Scotti Neuroradiology Unit, Humanitas Teaching Hospital, Rozzano, Milano, Italy

Neuroradiology Service, Humanitas Teaching Hospital, Rozzano, Milano, Italy

Timothy R. Smith Department of Neurosurgery, Brigham and Women's Hospital, Harvard Medical School, Boston, MA, USA

Valentina Vicennati Division of Endocrinology, Department of Medical and Surgical Science, Centre for Applied Biomedical Research (C.R.B.A.), S. Orsola-Malpighi Hospital, University of Bologna, Bologna, Italy

Craniopharyngiomas: Natural History and Clinical Presentation

1

Niki Karavitaki

Abstract

Craniopharyngiomas are rare epithelial tumours arising along the path of the craniopharyngeal duct and account for 2–5 % of all the primary intracranial neoplasms and for up to 15 % of the intracranial tumours in children. The majority (94–95 %) has a suprasellar component. The potential proximity to and the subsequent pressure effects of craniopharyngiomas on vital structures of the brain (visual pathways, brain parenchyma, ventricular system, major blood vessels and hypothalamo-pituitary system) predispose the patients to multiple clinical manifestations, the severity of which depends on the location, the size and the growth potential of the tumour. Headaches, nausea/vomiting, visual disturbances, growth failure (in children) and hypogonadism (in adults) are the most frequently reported. The hypothalamo-pituitary function at presentation may be severely affected and based on various series, GH deficiency is present in 35–100 % of the evaluated patients, FSH/LH deficiency in 38–91 %, ACTH deficiency in 21–68 %, TSH deficiency in 20–42 % and diabetes insipidus in 6–38 %. Early diagnosis is of major importance.

N. Karavitaki, MSc, PhD, FRCP
Institute of Metabolism and Systems Research, College of Medical and Dental Sciences, University of Birmingham, IBR Tower, Level 2, Birmingham, B15 2TT, UK

Centre for Endocrinology, Diabetes and Metabolism, Birmingham Health Partners, Birmingham, UK
e-mail: n.karavitaki@bham.ac.uk

© Springer International Publishing Switzerland 2016
A. Lania et al. (eds.), *Diagnosis and Management of Craniopharyngiomas: Key Current Topics*, DOI 10.1007/978-3-319-22297-4_1

1.1 Introduction

Craniopharyngiomas are rare epithelial tumours arising along the path of the cranio-pharyngeal duct, the canal connecting the stomodeal ectoderm with the evaginated Rathke's pouch. They may be diagnosed during childhood or adult life and are often associated with an enigmatic and unpredictable growth pattern, making their optimal management a subject of debate. Despite their benign histological appearance, their often infiltrative tendency into critical parasellar structures and their aggressive behaviour may result in significant morbidity and mortality (even after apparently successful therapy), posing a considerable medical and social problem.

1.2 History

Zenker in 1857 was the first to identify masses of cells resembling squamous epithelium along the pars distalis and pars tuberalis of the pituitary (Raimondi and Rougerie 1994). Extensive study of the squamous epithelial cells in the adenohypophysis followed in 1860 by H. Luschka, but the significance of these findings was not initially recognized, and for many decades, they remained overlooked (Karavitaki et al. 2006). In 1902, Fr. Saxer reported a tumour consisting of these cells (Karavitaki et al. 2006). Two years later, J. Erdheim, after a systematic study of the squamous epithelial cells in the adenohypophysis, described them only in the glands of adult patients, usually on the anterior surface of the infundibulum and in groups or islets of variable size, shape and number (Banna 1976). As a few of these groups of cells contained small cysts similar to some pituitary tumours unnamed at that time, he was convinced that both lesions had the same origin and called them hypophyseal duct neoplasms. Similar observations on clumps of cell rests were later published by Duffy, Kiyono and Carmichael (Karavitaki et al. 2006), but it was only in 1932 when squamous epithelial cells were also detected in the pituitary glands of childhood populations by W. Susman (1932). The first attempt for surgical removal of such a tumour ("from a patient presenting the symptoms associated with hypophyseal growths but without acromegaly") by Dr. Halstead in St. Luke's Hospital (Chicago) was reported in 1910 (Roderick et al. 2008). During the following years, different terminologies were used for them (including hypophyseal duct or craniopharyngeal duct or Rathke's pouch tumours, interpeduncular or dysontogenetic or suprasellar or craniobuccal cysts, suprasellar epitheliomas and adamantinomas), until in 1932 when the name "craniopharyngioma" was introduced by H. Cushing (Karavitaki et al. 2006).

1.3 Epidemiology

Craniopharyngiomas account for 2–5 % of all the primary intracranial neoplasms and for up to 15 % of the intracranial tumours in children (Karavitaki et al. 2006). Their incidence is reported as 0.13 per 100,000 person-years (Bunin et al. 1998), and genetic susceptibility seems unlikely. Craniopharyngiomas may be detected at any age, even in the prenatal and neonatal periods (Bailey et al. 1990; Müller-Scholden et al. 2000), and a bimodal age distribution with peak incidence rates of ages 5–14 and 50–74 years has been proposed (Bunin et al. 1998). In population-based studies from the USA and Finland, no gender differences have been found (Bunin et al. 1998; Sorva and Heiskanen 1986).

1.4 Presentation (Clinical and Hormonal Manifestations)

Craniopharyngiomas may arise anywhere along the craniopharyngeal canal, but most of them are located in the sellar/parasellar region. The majority (94–95 %) has a suprasellar component (purely suprasellar 20–41%/both supra- and intrasellar 53–75 %), whereas the purely intrasellar ones represent the least common variety (5–6 %) (Petito et al. 1976; Karavitaki et al. 2005). Occasionally, a suprasellar tumour may extend into the anterior (9 %), middle (8 %) or posterior (12 %) fossa (Petito et al. 1976). Other rare locations include the nasopharynx, the paranasal area, the sphenoid bone, the ethmoid sinus, the intrachiasmatic area, the temporal lobe, the pineal gland, the posterior cranial fossa, the cerebellopontine angle, the midportion of the midbrain or completely within the third ventricle (Karavitaki et al. 2006).

The potential proximity to and the subsequent pressure effects of craniopharyngiomas on vital structures of the brain (visual pathways, brain parenchyma, ventricular system, major blood vessels and hypothalamo-pituitary system) predispose the patients to multiple clinical manifestations, the severity of which depends on the location, the size and the growth potential of the tumour (Petito et al. 1976; Baskin and Wilson 1986; Weiner et al. 1994; Duff et al. 2000; Van Effenterre and Boch 2002; Karavitaki et al. 2005; Gautier et al. 2012; Nielsen et al. 2013). The duration of the symptoms until diagnosis ranges between 1 week and 372 months (Karavitaki et al. 2006). The commonest presenting clinical manifestations (neurological, visual, hypothalamo-pituitary) are summarized in Table 1.1.

Headaches, nausea/vomiting, visual disturbances, growth failure (in children) and hypogonadism (in adults) are the most frequently reported. Hydrocephalus

Table 1.1 Most frequent clinical manifestations of craniopharyngiomas in children and adults at presentation

Reference, number and age of patients	Headache	Nausea/vomiting	Papilloedema	Cranial nerve palsy	Ataxia/unsteadiness	Cognitive dysfunction[a]	Decreased consciousness/coma	Visual field defects
Petito et al. (1976) n=241	78 %	34 %	25 %			36 %		
Baskin and Wilson (1986) n=74 38<18 years	50 %							72 %
Hetelekides et al. (1993) n=61 All <21 years	77 %	43 %	29 %	20 %	18 %		3 %	
Weiner et al. (1994) n=56 26<19 years	7 % adults, 15 % children			8 % children		20 % adults, 8 % children		60 % adults, 54 % children
Duff et al. (2000) n=121 32≤16 years	74 %	21 %	10 %	2 %		10 %	29 %	62 %
Van Effenterre and Boch (2002) n=122 29<16 years	53 %		16 %	3 %		13 %	8 %	79 %
Karavitaki et al. (2005) n=119 41<16 years	56 % adults, 78 % children	26 % adults, 54 % children	6 % adults, 29 % children	9 % adults, 27 % children	3 % adults, 7 % children	17 % adults, 10 % children	4 % adults, 10 % children	60 % adults, 46 % children

Reference, number and age of patients	Decreased visual acuity or visual deterioration	Growth failure[b]	Failure of sexual development[b]	Hypogonadism (adults)	Poor energy	Somnolence	Anorexia/poor weight gain or weight loss	Obesity or weight gain	Polyuria/polydipsia
Gautier et al. (2012) n=171 65<18 years	61 % adults, 61 % children								46–79 %
Nielsen et al. (2013) n=189 39<15 years	59 % adults, 71.8 % children	17 % adults, 51.3 % children	7 % adults, 13 % children				13 % adults, 13 % children	3 % adults, 3 % children	
Range	7–81 %	21–54 %	6–29 %	2–27 %		3–18 %	8–36 %	3–29 %	46–79 %
Petito et al. (1976) n=241						20 %			6 %
Baskin and Wilson (1986) n=74 38<18 years		93 %		85 %					23 %
Hetelekides et al. (1993) n=61 All <21 years		25 %							13 %
Weiner et al. (1994) n=56 26<19 years	47 % adults, 50 % children	8 %	4 %	10 %				4 % children	3 % adults

(continued)

Table 1.1 (continued)

Reference, number and age of patients	Decreased visual acuity or visual deterioration	Growth failure[b]	Failure of sexual development[b]	Hypogonadism (adults)	Poor energy	Somnolence	Anorexia/poor weight gain or weight loss	Obesity or weight gain	Polyuria/polydipsia
Duff et al. (2000) n=121 32≤16 years	62 %	17 %	14 %		23 %			8 %	12 %
Van Effenterre and Boch (2002) n=122 29<16 years	80 %	45 %		40 %					18 %
Karavitaki et al. (2005) n=119 41<16 years	40 % adults, 39 % children	32 %	24 %	28 %	32 % adults, 22 % children	10 % adults, 5 % children	8 % adults, 20 % children	13 % adults, 5 % children	15 % adults, 15 % children
Gautier et al. (2012) n=171 55<18 years	71 % adults, 75 % children								12 % adults, 14 % children
Nielsen et al. (2013) n=189 39<15 years	65 % adults, 49 % children				47 % adults, 31 % children		10 % adults, 10 % children	17 % adults, 8 % children	19 % adults, 10 % children
Range	39–80 %	8–93 %	4–24 %	10–85 %	22–47 %	5–20 %	8–20 %	4–17 %	3–23 %

[a]Memory loss, impaired concentration, confusion, disorientation
[b]Children

has been described more commonly in children (Van Effenterre and Boch 2002; Karavitaki et al. 2005; Rosenfeld et al. 2014). Visual field defects usually present as bitemporal hemianopia (in up to 49 % of the cases) (Baskin and Wilson 1986; Duff et al. 2000). Notably, temporal alterations of their pattern due to intermittent emptying of the cyst fluid into the ventricular system may occur (Chen et al. 2003). Other less common or rare features include motor disorders, as hemi- or monoparesis; seizures; psychiatric symptoms, as emotional lability, hallucinations and paranoid delusions; autonomic disturbances; precocious puberty; the syndrome of inappropriate secretion of antidiuretic hormone; chemical meningitis due to spontaneous cyst rupture; hearing loss; anosmia; nasal obstruction; epistaxis; photophobia; emaciation, Weber's syndrome (ipsilateral III cranial nerve palsy with contralateral hemiplegia due to midbrain infarction); and Wallenberg's syndrome (signs due to occlusion of the posterior inferior cerebellar artery) (Karavitaki et al. 2006).

In a large series of patients comparing the presenting manifestations between childhood and adult populations, apart from headaches, nausea/vomiting, papilloedema and cranial nerve palsies, which were more frequent in children (probably associated with the high rates of hydrocephalus in this age group), no further differences in the clinical picture, the symptoms duration and the rates of endocrine deficits were found (Karavitaki et al. 2005).

It has been proposed that in cases of craniopharyngioma diagnosed in childhood, compromised growth rate is already evident in early infancy, whereas an increase in the weight tends to present later and is a predictor of obesity (Müller et al. 2004).

The hypothalamo-pituitary function at presentation may be severely affected, and in a series of 122 patients, 85 % of them had 1–3 hormone deficits (Van Effenterre and Boch 2002). A summary of the results of various studies using different diagnostic tests and criteria shows that GH deficiency is present in 35–100 % of the evaluated patients, FSH/LH deficiency in 38–91 %, ACTH deficiency in 21–68 %, TSH deficiency in 20–42 % and diabetes insipidus in 6–38 % (Table 1.2).

The differential diagnosis includes other sellar or parasellar tumours (Rathke's cleft cyst, dermoid cyst, epidermoid cyst, pituitary adenoma, germinoma, hamartoma, suprasellar aneurysm, arachnoid cyst, suprasellar abscess, Langerhans cell histiocytosis, sarcoidosis, tuberculosis, hypothalamic or optic pathway glioma, meningioma) (Karavitaki et al. 2006), and early diagnosis is of major importance.

Table 1.2 Pituitary hormone deficits and hyperprolactinemia at presentation in adults and children with craniopharyngioma

Reference number and age of patients	GH deficiency	FSH/LH deficiency[a]	ACTH deficiency	TSH deficiency	Hyperprolactinemia	Diabetes insipidus
Thomsett et al. (1980) n=42 All ≤17.2 years	13/18 (72 %)	3/8 (38 %)	4/17 (24 %)	7/29 (24 %)		4/24 (17 %)
Baskin and Wilson (1986) n=74 38<18 years			18/74 (24 %)	31/74 (42 %)		8/74 (12 %)
Hetelekides et al. (1993) n=61 All <21 years	12/34 (35 %)		7/34 (21 %)	7/34 (21 %)		8/34 (23 %)
Paja et al. (1995) n=35 13<19 years	27/35 (77 %)	27/33 (82 %)	12/35 (34 %)	13/35 (37 %)	7/29 (24 %)	13/35 (38 %)
De Ville et al. (1996) n=75 All<16.3 years	13/15 (87 %)	3/6 (50 %)	16/50 (32 %)	20/62 (32 %)	12/37 (32 %)	22/75 (29 %)
Honegger et al. (1999) n=143 30<16 years	59/82 (72 %) 17/23 in children (74 %) (74 %)	96/143 (77 %) 10/11 in children (91 %)	45/143 (32 %) 8/30 in children (27 %)	35/143 (25 %) 6/30 in children (20 %)	59/143 (41 %) 5/30 in children (17 %)	23/143 (16 %) 3/30 in children (10 %)
Karavitaki et al. (2005) n=121 42<16 years	21/22 (95 %) 15/15 in children (100 %)	40/54 (74 %)[b]	40/65 (62 %) 15/22 in children (68 %)	29/81 (36 %) 7/28 in children (25 %)	24/44 (55 %)[b]	19/104 (18 %) 7/32 in children (22 %)

(continued)

Table 1.2 (continued)

Reference number and age of patients	GH deficiency	FSH/LH deficiency[a]	ACTH deficiency	TSH deficiency	Hyperprolactinemia	Diabetes insipidus
Nielsen et al. (2013)	23/45	89/109	40/123	31/121		20/131
n=189	(51 %)	(82 %)	(33 %)	(26 %)		(15 %)
39<15 years	in adults		in adults	in adults		in adults
	5/9		8/20	7/27		2/32
	(56 %)		(40 %)	(26 %)		(6 %)
	in children		in children	in children		in children
Range	35–100 %	38–91 %	21–68 %	20–42 %	17–55 %	6–38 %

Number of patients with the deficit/total number of patients tested and relevant percentages

[a]Prepubertal children were excluded from the evaluations

[b]Only adults were included in the evaluations

Conclusions

Craniopharyngiomas may present with multiple clinical manifestations related to their location and subsequent pressure effects on vital structures (visual pathways, brain parenchyma, ventricular system, major blood vessels and hypothalamo-pituitary system). Headaches, nausea/vomiting, visual disturbances, growth failure (in children) and hypogonadism (in adults) are the most frequently reported. One or more pituitary hormone deficits may be already present at the time of tumour detection in a significant number of patients necessitating early diagnosis and adequate treatment.

References

Banna M (1976) Craniopharyngioma: based on 160 cases. Br J Radiol 49:206–223

Bailey W, Freidenberg GR, James HE, Hesselink JR, Jones KL (1990) Prenatal diagnosis of a craniopharyngioma using ultrasonography and magnetic resonance imaging. Prenat Diagn 10(1):623–629

Baskin DS, Wilson CB (1986) Surgical management of craniopharyngiomas. J Neurosurg 65:22–27

Bunin GR, Surawicz TS, Witman PA, Preston-Martin S, Davis F, Bruner JM (1998) The descriptive epidemiology of craniopharyngioma. J Neurosurg 89:547–551

Chen C, Okera S, Davies PE, Selva D, Crompton JL (2003) Craniopharyngioma: a review of long-term visual outcome. Clin Experiment Ophthalmol 31:220–228

De Vile CJ, Grant DB, Hayward RD, Stanhope R (1996) Growth and endocrine sequelae of craniopharyngioma. Arch Dis Child 75:108–114

Duff JM, Meyer FB, Ilstrup DM, Laws ER Jr, Scleck CD, Scheithauer BW (2000) Long-term outcomes for surgically resected craniopharyngiomas. Neurosurgery 46(2):291–305

Gautier A, Godbout A, Grosheny C, Tejedor I, Coudert M, Courtillot C, Jublanc C, De Kerdanet M, Poirier JY, Riffaud L, Sainte-Rose C, Van Effenterre R, Brassier G, Bonnet F, Touraine P, Craniopharyngioma Study Group (2012) Markers of recurrence and long-term morbidity in craniopharyngioma: a systematic analysis of 171 patients. J Clin Endocrinol Metab 97(4):1258–1267

Hetelekidis S, Barnes PD, Tao ML, Fischer EG, Schneider L, Scott RM, Tarbell NJ (1993) 20-year experience in childhood craniopharyngioma. Int J Radiat Oncol Biol Phys 27:189–195

Honegger J, Buchfelder M, Fahlbusch R (1999) Surgical treatment of craniopharyngiomas: endocrinological results. J Neurosurg 90:251–257

Karavitaki N, Brufani C, Warner JT, Adams CB, Richards P, Ansorge O, Shine B, Turner HE, Wass JA (2005) Craniopharyngiomas in children and adults: systematic analysis of 121 cases with long-term follow-up. Clin Endocrinol (Oxf) 62:397–409

Karavitaki N, Cudlip S, Adams CB, Wass JA (2006) Craniopharyngiomas. Endocr Rev 27:371–397

Müller HL, Emser A, Faldum A, Bruhnken G, Etavard-Gorris N, Gebhardt U, Oeverink R, Kolb R, Sörensen N (2004) Longitudinal study on growth and body mass index before and after diagnosis of childhood craniopharyngioma. J Clin Endocrinol Metab 89(7):3298–3305

Müller-Scholden J, Lehrnbecker T, Müller HL, Bensch J, Hengen RH, Sörensen N, Stockhausen HB (2000) Radical surgery in a neonate with craniopharyngioma—report of a case. Pediatr Neurosurg 33:265–269

Nielsen EH, Jørgensen JO, Bjerre P, Andersen M, Andersen C, Feldt-Rasmussen U, Poulsgaard L, Kristensen LO, Astrup J, Jørgensen J, Laurberg P (2013) Acute presentation of craniopharyngioma in children and adults in a Danish national cohort. Pituitary 16:528–535

Paja M, Lucas T, Garcia-Uria F, Salame F, Barcelo B, Estrada J (1995) Hypothalamic-pituitary dysfunction in patients with craniopharyngioma. Clin Endocrinol 42:467–473

Petito CK, De Girolami U, Earle K (1976) Craniopharyngiomas. A clinical and pathological review. Cancer 37:1944–1952

Raimondi AJ, Rougerie J (1994) A critical review of personal experiences with craniopharyngioma: clinical history, surgical technique and operative results. Pediatr Neurosurg 21:134–150

Roderick E, Karavitaki N, Wass JA (2008) Craniopharyngiomas. Historical aspects on their management. Hormones 7(3):271–274

Rosenfeld A, Arrington D, Miller J, Olson M, Gieseking A, Etzl M, Harel B, Schembri A, Kaplan A (2014) A review of childhood and adolescent craniopharyngiomas with particular attention to hypothalamic obesity. Pediatr Neurol 50(1):4–10

Sorva R, Heiskanen O (1986) Craniopharyngioma in Finland. A study of 123 cases. Acta Neurochir (Wien) 81(3–4):85–89

Susman W (1932) Embryonic epithelial rests in the pituitary. Br J Surg 19:571–576

Thomsett MJ, Conte FA, Kaplan SL, Grumbach MM (1980) Endocrine and neurologic outcome in childhood craniopharyngioma: review of effect of treatment in 42 patients. J Pediatr 97:728–735

Van Effenterre R, Boch AL (2002) Craniopharyngioma in adults and children: a study of 122 surgical cases. J Neurosurg 97:3–11

Weiner HL, Wisoff JH, Rosenberg ME, Kupersmith MJ, Cohen H, Zagzag D, Shiminski-Maher T, Flamm ES, Epsten FJ, Miller D (1994) Craniopharyngiomas: a clinicopathological analysis of factors predictive of recurrence and functional outcome. Neurosurgery 35(6):1001–1011

Craniopharyngioma: Pathological and Molecular Aspects

Federico Roncaroli and Juan Pedro Martinez-Barbera

Abstract

Craniopharyngioma (CP) (ICD-O 9350/1) is defined as a benign, partly cystic, epithelial tumour presumably derived from the Rathke's pouch epithelium. CPs are classified in two forms with distinct morphological and molecular features: adamantinous (ACP) (ICD-O 9351/1) and papillary CP (PCP) (ICD-O 9352/1). Both ACP and PCP are regarded as grade I lesions by the World Health Organisation (WHO) Classification of Tumours of the Central Nervous System (CNS) (Rushing et al., Craniopharyngioma. In: Louis DN, Ohgaki H, Wiestler OD, Webster KC (eds) WHO classification of tumours of the central nervous system, 3rd edn. World Health Organization Press, Geneva, Switzerland, pp. 238–240, 2007). Rare tumours with mixed features of ACP and PCP have been described (Okada et al. 2010; Prieto and Pascual 2013). In this chapter, the pathological features of craniopharyngiomas as well as the latest results of molecular studies will be discussed.

2.1 An Historical Note

We owe the Austrian pathologist Jakob Erdheim (1874–1937) the first systematic description of CP with the publication of his pioneer study in 1904. Whilst conducting the post-mortem of an elderly woman in 1902, Erdheim observed a

F. Roncaroli (✉)
Institute of Brain, Behaviour and Mental Health, The University of Manchester, UK
e-mail: federico.roncaroli@manchester.ac.uk

J.P. Martinez-Barbera
Birth Defects Research Centre, UCL Institute of Child Health, London, UK
e-mail: j.martinez-barbera@ucl.ac.uk

© Springer International Publishing Switzerland 2016
A. Lania et al. (eds.), *Diagnosis and Management of Craniopharyngiomas: Key Current Topics*, DOI 10.1007/978-3-319-22297-4_2

cyst on the anterior surface of the pituitary gland that was lined with cuboidal, squamous and ciliated epithelium. He noted the cyst was different from the small cysts derived from the Rathke's pouch, which often lie between the anterior and posterior lobe. Interested in such finding and almost certainly unaware of the 1860 Herbert Luschka's extensive work documenting adenohypophyseal squamous epithelial cells that are similar to the oral mucosa, Erdheim set out to examine the glands from 13 adults and six newborns. He found similar squamous nests in ten adults but not in the newborns. Erdheim published his results in a ponderous manuscript that lucidly illustrated the findings. From the description, it appears that five cases could have been CPs. He subsequently searched the well-organised records and specimen archives of the Institute of Pathology at the Vienna General Hospital for sellar and parasellar tumours that contained similar nests and small islands squamous epithelium (Fig. 2.1). He found seven such cases documented between 1828 and 1889.

Erdheim knew from the observation of the German zoologist Martin Heinrich Rathke in 1838 that the adenohypophysis arises from the hypophysial duct, the cranial part of which grows into developing the pouch of ectodermal epithelium from the stomodeum. Erdheim proposed that CPs could have been derived from sequestered squamous epithelium and defined the lesion as tumours of the hypophysial duct. Erdheim's pathogenetic theory encountered a large consensus despite of the fact that squamous cell nests are only occasionally observed in children (Hunter

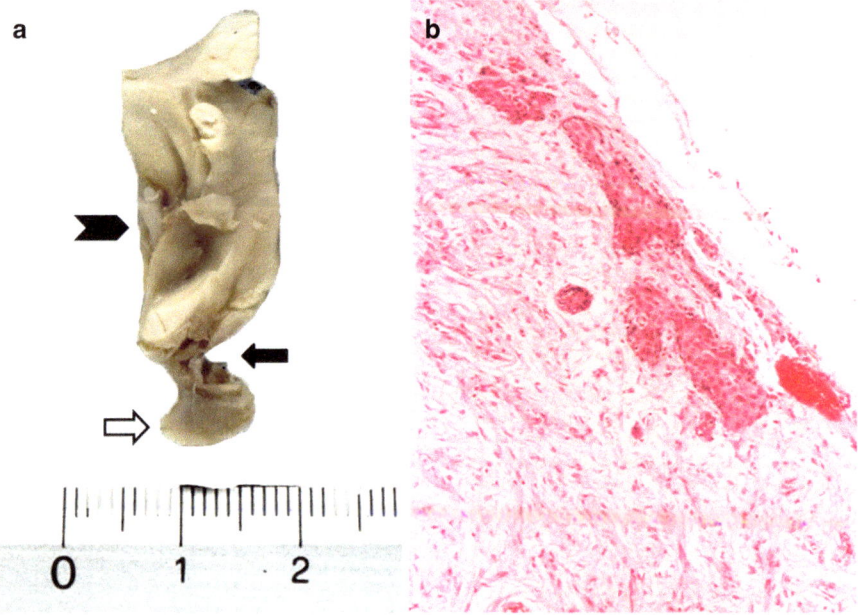

Fig. 2.1 (a) Sagittal anatomical preparation of post-mortem adenohypophysis (*white arrow*), infundibulum (*dark arrow*) and hypothalamus (*arrowhead*); (b) nests of squamous epithelium are present in the infundibulum (HE, ×20)

1955; Goldberg and Eshbaugh 1960) and the hypophyseal duct is lined by cuboidal rather than squamous epithelium. The possibility of squamous metaplasia of gonadotroph and corticotroph cells in the *pars tuberalis* was also suggested as an alternative theory.

Erdheim was also aware of the variation in the histology of CPs and noted that a considerable proportion of cases resembled ameloblastoma. Erroneous but in line with Rudolph Virchow's belief and the general opinion of the time that all large tumours in the sella were aggressive, Jakob Erdheim claimed that a high proportion of CPs were malignant.

Several accounts in the literature preceded Erdheim's seminal work. The first description of a putative CP could probably be attributed to Friedrich Albert von Zenker in 1857 who depicted a cystic suprasellar mass containing cholesterol crystals and squamous epithelium found at autopsy, whilst the first detailed report of what seems a PCP was given by Mott and Barrett in 1899 (Mott and Barrett 1899). The clinical manifestation of CP was first described by Boyce and Beadles in 1893 when documenting a 35-year-old blind patient who fell in coma and died as a result of a large, partially ossified cystic lesion, which caused brainstem, optic chiasm and optic tract compression.

The exhaustive review published by Critchley and Ironside in 1926 is certainly worth reading for the critical account given by the authors of the early discussion of the origin of the disease and the related terminology (Critchley and Ironside 1926).

During the years that followed Erdheim's work, the disease was defined with different terminologies until the term CP was coined by Charles Frazier in 1931 (Frazier and Alpers 1931) and subsequently popularised by Harvey Cushing in the report of his series of brain tumours published in 1932 (Cushing 1932). Although craniopharyngeal duct and CP are inaccurate terms and the correct name for the duct would in fact be craniobuccal duct, Cushing's words 'this admittedly somewhat cumbersome term has been employed, for want of something more brief to include the kaleidoscopic tumours, solid and cystic, which take their origin from epithelial rests ascribable to an imperfect closure of the hypophysial or craniopharyngeal duct' (Cushing 1932) somehow marked the beginning of the history of one the diseases whose management has probably caused more debate and disagreement than any other between endocrinologists, neurosurgeons and oncologists.

The history of craniopharyngioma has extensively and elegantly been reviewed in the following studies: Lindholm and Nielsen (2009), Barkhoudarian and Laws (2013) and Pascual et al. (2015).

2.2 Adamantinous Craniopharyngioma

ACP is defined as a sellar and suprasellar neoplasm with features resembling ameloblastoma or keratinising and calcifying odontogenic cyst (Rushing et al. 2007). The word 'adamantinous' derives from the ancient Greek word 'αδαμας', which defines the hardness of stone (Critchley and Ironside 1926) and emphasises one of the hallmarks of ACP: calcification.

2.2.1 Macroscopic Features

Adamantinous CP usually presents as a firm and often calcified, lobulated, partially cystic lesion with an average size of 3–4 cm. Adamantinous CPs almost always extend to the suprasellar compartment. Purely intrasellar and purely suprasellar examples are considerably less common (Petito et al. 1976; Karavitaki et al. 2005). Large tumours can rarely reach to the anterior, middle or posterior fossa. Adamantinous CPs characteristically adhere to the stalk, adenohypophysis, hypothalamus, vessels and nerves, and they frequently cause indentation of the floor of the III ventricle. Recurrent tumours tend to be more adherent than the primary lesions. The cyst is typically filled with turbid, dense, dark brown fluid reminiscent of motor oil that contains crystals of cholesterol resulting from desquamated keratin within the cavity. Crystals can easily be visualised by smearing the fluid on a glass slides and examining the specimen under polarised light (Fig. 2.2). Though common of ACP, cholesterol crystals can be found in other sellar lesions such as inflamed or haemorrhagic Rathke's clef cysts and sellar xanthogranuloma (Sumida et al. 1994).

2.2.2 Microscopic Features

Histological features of ACP are distinctive (Rushing et al. 2007; Larkin and Ansorge 2013). ACP typically shows solid and cystic components. Solid areas have lobular architecture with lobules reminiscent of clover leafs and composed of

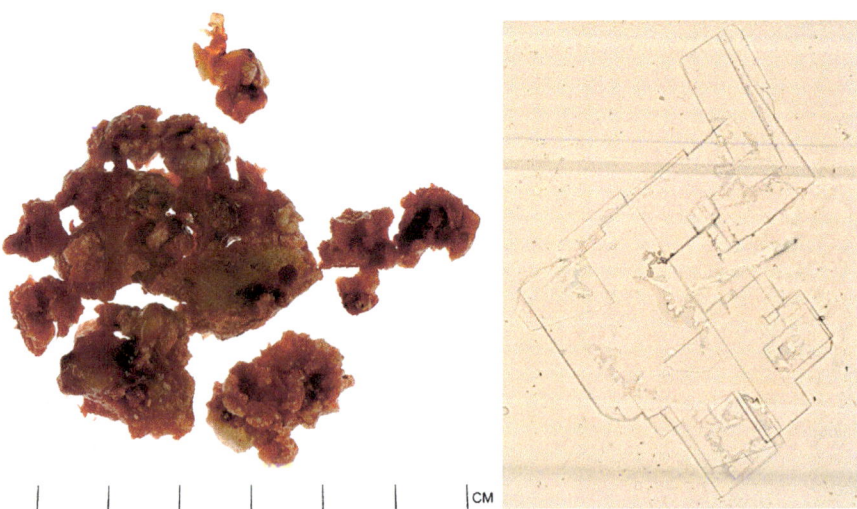

Fig. 2.2 Macroscopically, adamantinous craniopharyngioma appears as brown, friable tissue (*left* – Courtesy of Dr. Ann Sandison, Imperial College, London); cyst content contains cholesterol crystals that can be visualised by simply smearing the fluid on a glass slide (*right*, unstained smear – ×40)

anastomosing trabeculae of pseudostratified columnar cells. Neoplastic cells at the periphery of lobules line to form palisades, whilst loose-textured aggregates of discohesive, stellate cells characterise the inner portion of lobules. Tumour cells are uniform. Overt nuclear atypia and pleomorphism are uncommon. Sudden keratinisation is the norm and consists of nodules and eosinophilic, anucleated, keratinised ghost cells, broadly known as 'wet keratin'. Wet keratin may undergo calcification. Cyst spaces result from degeneration of keratin nodules and are filled with cell debris or fluid. Cells lining larger cysts are often flattened and resemble the lining of keratinous cyst or PCP, but unlike epidermoid cysts, keratohyalin granules and thin, anucleated squames are absent (Fig. 2.3a–c).

In addition to the epithelial components, ACP often shows extensive fibrosis, chronic inflammation, haemosiderin deposits and cholesterol clefts (Fig. 2.3d). These changes and particularly calcification can be extensive and obscure the epithelial component in recurrent tumours and in ACPs after intracavital treatment (Szeifert et al. 1990) so that identification of wet keratin remains the only diagnostic clue. Granulomas associated with cholesterol clefts and giant cells

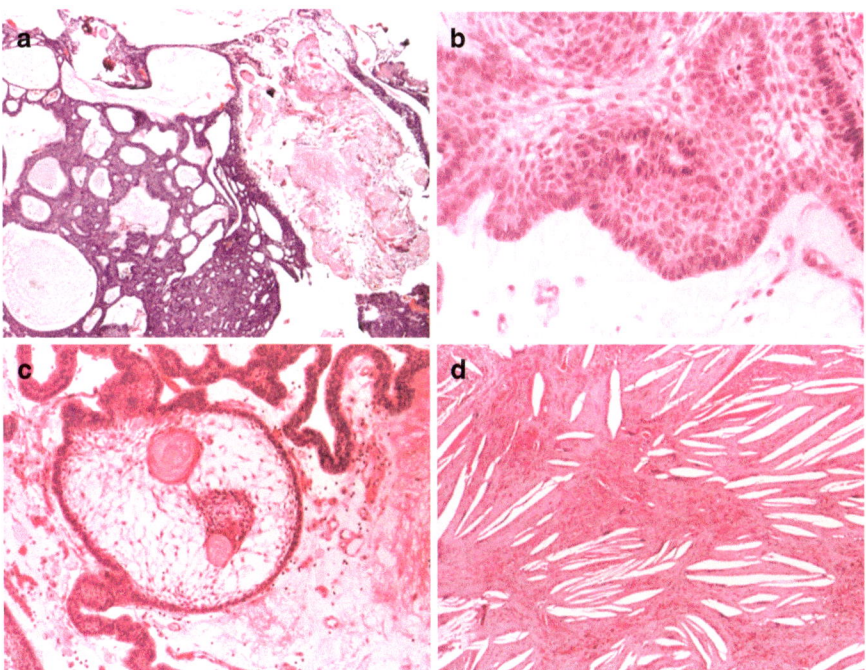

Fig. 2.3 Histologically, adamantinous craniopharyngioma is characterised by anastomosing trabeculae of and clover leaf-like epithelial lobules lined by layers of pseudostratified columnar cells that forms palisades around loose aggregates of stellate cells; abrupt keratinisation is a constant feature of adamantinous craniopharyngioma (**a**, HE – ×4). Neoplastic cells show variable amount of cytoplasm and rounded to spindle, hyperchromatic nucleus (**b**, HE – ×20); the stroma is loose and contains stellate cells (**c**, HE – ×10); cystic spaces contain haemorrhagic fluid with cholesterol crystals (**d**, HE – ×10)

can occasionally be seen. Melanin pigment is rare but described in ACP (Harris et al. 1999). Exceptionally ACPs may contain teeth (Seemayer et al. 1972; Beaty and Ahn 2014).

All these features are pathognomonic of ACP and absent in PCP.

The similarities between ACP and some odontogenic tumours have long been established given their common origin from the oral ectoderm (Bernstein and Buchino 1997). Morphological and genetic similarities between ACP and amelo-blastoma and keratinising and calcifying odontogenic cyst have been extensively described. In the study of 54 APCs, Paulus and colleagues documented features similar to calcifying odontogenic cyst in 50 % ACP (Paulus et al. 1997), to amelo-blastoma in 24 % and hybrid morphology in 15 %. Other similarities between odontogenic lesions and ACP include the expression of enamel proteins such as enamelin and amelogenin and the proteinase enamelysin and tooth formation (Beaty and Ahn 2014). ACP and calcifying odontogenic cyst show mutations in *CTNNB1* gene and nuclear accumulation of β-catenin. Notably, enamel proteins have not been found in PCPs.

2.2.3 Electron Microscopy

Ultrastructural features of ACP include well-formed desmosomes connecting epi-thelial cells, tonofilaments in bundles or lying randomly and basal lamina where epithelial cells form palisades. Cells that line cyst lack basal lamina and have micro-villi (Ghatak et al. 1971).

2.3 Papillary Craniopharyngioma

Papillary CP is defined as a well-differentiated pseudopapillary epithelial neoplasm of the sellar and suprasellar region (Rushing et al. 2007).

The first detailed description of PCP is due to Giangaspero et al. (1984), who reported six adult cases of suprasellar CPs that were characterised by solid rather than cystic structure, well-differentiated papillary squamous epithelium without calcification, palisaded cells or nodules of 'wet' keratin.

2.3.1 Macroscopic Features

Papillary craniopharyngiomas tend to be smaller than ACP with a reported mean size of 2.6 cm. They are rarely calcified; more commonly predominantly solid though pure solid examples are rare. PCPs are usually better circumscribed and less adhesive to surrounding structures than ACP. When cystic, the cyst content is clear, often described as viscous and yellow, and does not contain cholesterol crys-tals. In some cystic PCPs, the cyst may be large relative to the size of the nodule. In mixed solid and cystic tumours, the solid component typically consisted of a small (often less than 1 cm), yellow–green mural nodule. Location is similar to ACP although PCP is more often suprasellar, and it can be confined to the third ventricle (Crotty et al. 1995).

2.3.2 Microscopic Features

Histologically, PCP is composed of sheets of well-differentiated squamous epithelial cells centred by fibrovascular stroma. Sheets tend to dehisce to form the pseudopapillae that are characteristic of the lesion. The basal cell layer may show some palisading, but this feature is never as prominent as ACP. Small aggregates or whorls of keratinised cells can be seen in some tumours but never in the form of flaky keratin or nodules of 'wet' keratin. The epithelium lining cysts can be focally attenuated and lack pseudopapillae closely resembling RCC with squamous metaplasia (Fig. 2.4a–c). Small groups or single goblet cells within the squamous epithelium are present in about one-third of PCPs. Ciliated cells are less common being only seen in 4 % of tumours. Goblet or ciliated cells in PCP are similar to those seen in RCC. In such instances, the differential diagnosis between PCP and RCC with abundant squamous metaplasia can be challenging (Matsushima et al. 1980; Oka et al. 1997; Crotty et al. 1995).

The stroma of PCP often contains small aggregates of lymphocytes and plasma cells and, in some instances, foamy macrophages. Stroma can at times appear hypocellular and hyalinised. Stellate cells that are typical of ACP are lacking. Secondary changes such as haemorrhages, necrosis and microcalcification are uncommon. Rare CPs can show mixed features of ACP and PCP either appearing as alternating components or exceptionally as intermediate appearance (Crotty et al. 1995; Okada et al. 2010; Prieto and Pascual 2013).

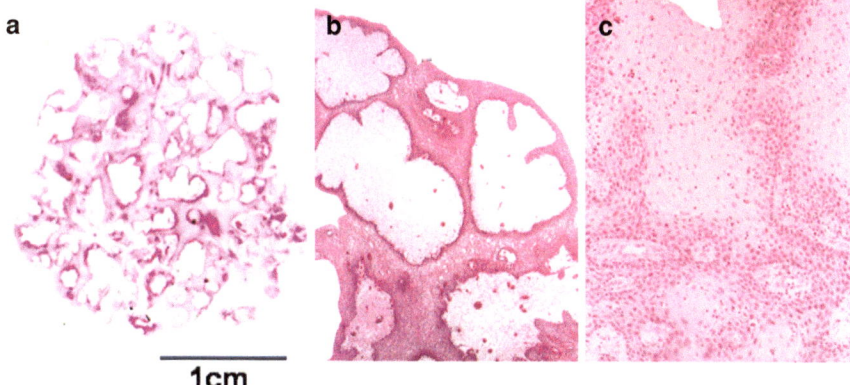

Fig. 2.4 Papillary craniopharyngioma usually presents as a rounded, well-circumscribed lesion (**a**, HE – whole mount) and consists of sheets of remarkably well-differentiated squamous epithelial cells growing around cores of fibrovascular stroma (**b**, HE – ×4). Away from the surface, neoplastic cells show typical squamoid differentiation (**c**, HE – ×20). No wet keratin is present

2.3.3 Electron Microscopy

Ultrastructural features of epithelial cells in PCP are not dissimilar to APC. The cytoplasm contains abundant bundles of tonofilaments. Cell-to-cell junctions consist of well-formed desmosomes, and surface cell may show prominent microvilli (Crotty et al. 1995).

2.4 The Immunoprofile of Craniopharyngioma

The histopathological features of ACP are straightforward, and the diagnosis does not usually require any immunohistochemical stains. Nevertheless, Szeifert and colleagues (1990) observed that over 20 % of surgical samples do not contain enough material for correct assessment. The diagnosis can be particularly challenging when ACPs are predominantly cystic and the tissue comes from the fenestration of the wall or APCs that are entirely suprasellar and therefore difficult to access surgically. In such cases, immunostains for cytokeratins may help to identify isolated neoplastic cells. Papillary CPs can more often be misdiagnosed on small biopsies.

The cytokeratin profile of CPs has been investigated in a few studies. Asa and colleagues (1981) first reported that cytokeratins are present in the surface epithelium of ACP but not by neoplastic stellate, stromal cells but this study did not distinguish between the various cytokeratin isoforms. More recently, Tateyama and colleagues (2001) gave a more detailed account of cytokeratin expression and found that CPs are positive for the cocktail of high molecular weight cytokeratin AE1/AE3. In ACPs, cytokeratin 7 is stronger in stellate and squamous cells than in palisading columnar cells, whilst PCPs mainly show cytokeratin 7 in the superficial layer of stratified squamous epithelium. Cytokeratin 8 is consistently positive in ACPs but not all PCPs. When positive, cytokeratin 8 is expressed in the superficial epithelial layer. Immunolabelling for cytokeratin 14 is strong and diffuse, and human hair keratin is only present in the shadow cells of ACPs. Kurosaki and colleagues (2001) looked at the best cytokeratin to diagnose CP in small biopsies and when no obvious epithelium is present. Cytokeratins were demonstrated in over 92 % of cases, but the number of positive cells and intensity of immunostain varied among the lesions. Cytokeratins 7 and 19 were found in 50–100 % of cells, and their distribution and intensity were similar. In contrast, the distribution of cytokeratin 7 differed from keratin M-903 as the outer palisaded basal layer was intensely positive for seven in only half of cases. Papillary CP showed moderate staining with cytokeratin 7 in the superficial cell layer, whereas basal or midzone epithelial cells were negative. The basal layer was also negative for 19.

Similar to pilomatrixoma and calcifying odontogenic tumour and cyst, the 38-kDa type-1 transmembrane sialomucin-like glycoprotein podoplanin is expressed in shadow cells of ACPs but not in PCPs, whilst hard α-keratin was found mainly in epithelial cells of the stratum intermedium of some ACPs and predominantly in marginal basaloid cells of PCPs (Kusama et al. 2005; Kikuchi et al. 2012).

Craniopharyngiomas can express oestrogen receptor though at variable levels and often in a minority of tumour cells. Using in situ hybridisation study, Thapar et al. (1994) found the transcript in 15 ACPs and four PCP, but only two lesions reportedly expressed the protein. Progesterone receptor gene expression has been reported by Honegger et al. (1997), but it is unclear whether the receptor is active. Interestingly, Elmaci and colleagues (2002) found intense progesterone receptor expression in their case of PCP that metastasised to the left frontotemporal lobe.

Aside from the discovery of β-catenin mutations in ACPs that result in translocation of the protein to the nucleus, some studies have suggested the use of β-catenin immunostaining to differentiate between ACPs and other interstellar, nonadenomatous tumours (Hofmann et al. 2006). The immunostain for mutant protein BRAFV600E is conversely used in the differential diagnosis between PCP and Rathke's clef cyst (Schweizer et al. 2014).

A study tested p63 with immunohistochemistry and qPCR (Cao et al. 2010) and found protein overexpression in 45 out of 51 ACPs and 14 out of 15 PCPs. P63 stained the basal layer cells and the whorl-like arrays ACPs and was uniform in PCPs. No correlation was found between p63 and Ki-67 stained. Similar gene expression was observed when comparing the five cases with high p63 versus normal tissue, with decreasing transcript of TAp63 mRNA and increasing DNp63 mRNA.

ACPs show low to absent immunoreactivity for MGMT (Zuhur et al. 2011), but no studies on MGMT methylation have been published so far and no studies have correlated MGMT status to resistance to alkylating agents.

SOX2 and OCT4 are embryonic stem cell markers known to be expressed in the marginal zone of the human pituitary in the so-called pituitary stem/progenitor cell niche. In contrast, KL4 and NANOG were never been investigated in such location. Two studies examined stem cell markers in CPs. With the hypothesis that CPs may be derived from postnatal pituitary stem cells rather than the Rathke's pouch or metaplastic cells in the pituitary stalk, Garcia-Lavandeira and colleagues (2012) studied the expression of stem cell markers in a series of 20 CPs including 18 APCs and two PCPs. Irrespective of the type, CPs expressed SOX2, OCT4 and KLF4. SOX2 and OCT4 were found to be limited to the nuclei of basal cells with the expression fading in the stellate or squamous cells. KLF4 and SOX9 showed more diffuse pattern in the three epithelial layers of AC. In PCP, SOX2, OCT4, KLF4 and SOX9 were mainly seen in the nuclei of basal epithelial cells and with a lower intensity towards the surface. Five APCs were positive for RET and GFRA3. RET expression was intense in the basal cell layer surrounding the cysts, whilst GFRA3 was expressed in the stellate cells. More recently, Holsken and colleagues (2014) observed frequent expression of prominin (CD133) in the basal cell layer of ACPs but not PCPs, whereas CD44 expression was widespread to PCPs and only restricted to a few cells in ACPs. Holsken's study further proves the existence of a stem cell phenotype in CPs.

2.5 Can Pathology Predict Recurrence?

Although CP is classified as WHO grade I lesion, ACPs and PCPs can cause significant morbidity due to their vicinity to hypothalamus, pituitary gland and optic chiasm. Despite the homogenous histological features, the biological behaviour of CPs varies considerably among patients. Overall, it is reported that up to over 40 % of CPs recur within 1–3 years from surgery (Prieto et al. 2013; Hussain et al. 2013; Müller 2014). Disease-related death can even occur many years after treatment due to multiple recurrences, chronic hypothalamic insufficiency, hormonal deficiencies, cerebrovascular disease and seizures (reviewed in Erfurth et al. 2013; Müller 2014). Whether or not the size of CP has impact on patients outcome is controversial, though one study showed increased survival rates in patients with a CP smaller than 3 cm (reviewed in Prieto et al. 2013), and even CPs that are totally resected can recur in up to 50 % of patients (reviewed in Hussain et al. 2013). Also, the interval between surgery and relapse is unpredictable. As said, the proximity of CP to vital structures is a major challenge to achieving a cure, and the key question is to identify the best candidates for a radical versus conservative treatment. Several clinical multinational cooperative studies have addressed this question. Less invasive approaches have gained credit and led to the need to identifying histopathological features on small biopsies that can predict the short- and long-term outcomes. The pathological features that associate with a higher recurrence risk or rapid regrowth have not yet been clearly defined, and the knowledge of the underlying factors for a CP's aggressive behaviour is very limited and mostly based on single cases. For this reason, the search of tissue biomarkers of recurrences at pathological examination has attracted several investigators (Gupta et al. 2006; Gautier et al. 2012).

To help clarifying such factors, Prieto and colleagues (2013) comprehensively reviewed 52 studies including series and single case reports that looked at the factors influencing and predicting recurrence in CPs. Their work faced the difficulty residing in the heterogeneity of epidemiological data and of the topographic and pathological definition of extent tumour removal as well as the heterogeneity of surgical features documented in the various studies. The concept itself of recurrence varied among authors with some using the term relapse as the regrowth of a totally removed CP and others including those tumours that grew back from a post-surgical residue.

The evaluation of Ki-67 labelling index produced inconsistent results in predicting tumour regrowth. In fact, the results of studies that investigated cell proliferation using Ki-67 alone or in association with other makers such as cyclin (Losa et al. 2004), p53 (Tena-Suck et al. 2006) or PCNA (Kayaselçuk et al. 2002) were controversial with some authors documenting a positive correlation with outcome (Nishi et al. 1999; Izumoto et al. 2005) and others failing to prove any predictive value (Raghavan et al. 2000; Agozzino et al. 2006; Kim et al. 2001; Duò et al. 2003; Losa et al. 2004). The reported cut-off of Ki-67-positive cells varied broadly among studies with a range between 0.1 and 49 %. Nishi and colleagues (Nishi et al. 1999) suggested a cut-off of 7 %, but their proposal has not been validated by subsequent studies. The uneven distribution of positive cells is a factor that affects the correlation with outcomes, particularly when small tissue is available. Nevertheless, in clinical practice and when dealing with single cases, a high Ki-67 in the primary tumour should be taken into consideration as possible indicator of a more aggressive behaviour and tendency to rapidly recur (Prieto et al. 2013). Proliferation is always high in malignant Cps (Sofela et al. 2014). Markers of cell proliferation other than Ki-67 such as the 3H-thymidine incorporation (Broggi et al. 1994), minichromosome maintenance protein 6 and DNA topoisomerase II alpha (Xu et al. 2007) reportedly correlated with outcome, thus supporting the idea that a high cell proliferation impacts on CP recurrence.

Similar contradictory results were obtained when p53 expression was compared to outcome. One study proposed p53 to be predictive of high risk of recurrence (Tena-Suck et al. 2006), and one study observed a high p53 in the recurrent compared to the primary tumour (Prieto et al. 2013).

The consistency of CP and the extent of the cystic component may also influence the extent of tumour removal and therefore the outcome, whilst others documented higher recurrence rates of mixed cystic and solid CPs compared with those predominantly cystic (Shapiro et al. 1979). In this respect, the expression of carbonic anhydrase IX (CA IX) and hypoxia-induced factor 1 alpha (HIF-1α) has been investigated as a possible mechanism of cyst formation (Proescholdt et al. 2011). CA IX was found in 85 % of CP and mostly of the adamantinous type, whilst only a minority of PCPs were positive. Expression of CA IX was found to be intense in the epithelial cell layer and palisading cells. HIF-1α staining was weak to absent although it is one of the main inductors of CA IX. Noticeable VEGF was only found in 30 % of cases, and no correlation was found between VEGF and CA IX. Ultrastructural analysis revealed fenestrations in the endothelium, a feature that can be induced by VEGF and may account for the increased vascular permeability leading to fluid leak and cyst formation. Active fluid production rather than leak has also been suggested. In fact, the evidence that cyst fluid in CP has low protein content, high lactate levels and low pH value suggests an active process rather than passive plasma efflux secondary to a leak of the blood–brain barrier breakdown. Interestingly these same authors documented different CA IX level in ACP and PCP.

The study of molecular prognostic indicators of recurrence has also demonstrated a number of gene expression patterns highlighting the difference between primary and recurrent CPs. Of these, recurrent CPs show increased platelet-derived growth factor receptor-α (PDGFR-α), fibroblast growth factor-2 (FGF-2) (reviewed in Hussain et al. 2013) and molecular determinants of angiogenesis.

Angiogenesis has attracted the attention of several groups. Formation of new vessels is a key requirement for tumour growth in order to allow oxygenation, nutrient perfusion and the removal of metabolic waste, and it undoubtedly favours recurrence. Studies have documented an increase in microvascular density (MVD) and vascular endothelial growth factor (VEGF) expression in recurrent tumours (Vidal et al. 2002). It is of note that VEGF and MVD are higher in recurrent ACPs than PCPs (Xu et al. 2006) and that β-catenin is a regulator of VEGF and likely responsible of mediating angiogenesis in ACPs. Studies focussed on MVD and expression of VEGF and its receptor to explain cyst formation and as predictors of recurrence.

Vaquero and colleagues (Vaquero et al. 1999) concentrated on cyst formation because cysts are often responsible of pressure on the surrounding structures, regardless of tumour size, and therefore a cause of morbidity. Of the 12 adult PCPs, four were predominantly solid and eight mostly cystic. VEGF expression was found to be variable but consistently weak to absent in the four solid tumours. In the cystic lesions, expression was localised in the squamous epithelial layer of the cyst wall.

Vidal et al. (2002) looked at VEGF in 22 ACPs and 10 PCPs and observed strong cytoplasmic immunolabelling in the epithelium of both tumour types, whereas the stroma was negative. VEGF immunostaining correlated with MVD, whilst no firm correlation was observed between MVD and patient age and gender, histotype or disease recurrence. Papillary CPs showed higher MVD than ACPs, probably reflecting the vascularisation of papillae. The authors detected VEGFR-2 mRNA in the epithelial and endothelial cells of both ACP and PCP but not in the connective tissue stroma. A positive correlation was also documented between the expression of VEGFR-2 mRNA and VEGF immunolabelling. They also found that highly vascularised CPs recurred irrespective of whether they were treated with surgery or radiotherapy following incomplete excision. In contrast, MVD was similar in recurrent and nonrecurrent lesions when subtotally removed. This result suggests poorly vascularised CPs recur more frequently if not treated with radiotherapy.

Xu and co-authors (2006) studied 32 ACPs, 31 PCPs and 20 recurrences and found significantly different expressions of VEGF and MVD between ACP and PCP but no significant difference in VEGF and MVD between primary and recurrent tumours and no difference between recurrence-free and recurrence patients in either subtype. VEGF was present in the cytoplasm of tumour cell nest and stroma of APCa, and the strongest staining was observed in vascular endothelial cells. In PCP, the staining of squamous epithelial cells was intense though the strongest immunolabelling was observed the microvessels.

Sun et al. (2010) investigated FGF-2, fibronectin, PDGF-A, PDGF-B, PDGFR-α and PDGFR-β and tested the angiogenic capacity of ten ACP (six nonrecurrent and four recurrent) in a corneal angiogenesis model. Their results showed that recurrent ACPs have significantly higher angiogenic potential than nonrecurrent tumours. FGF-2 was only expressed in recurrent CPs, whilst VEGF and fibronectin were found in both tumour types, and the levels of expression were similar for recurrent and nonrecurrent lesions.

Xia et al. (2011) tested MMP-9, VEGF and collagen IV and found significantly higher MMP-9 expression in the recurrent cases along with significantly increased VEGF. They also found disruption of the basal lamina in recurrent tumours when compared with the primary lesion.

Epithelial mesenchymal transition EMT seems to be relevant to the progression of ACP. Increase in vimentin and decreased E-cadherin were associated with recurrence and poor postoperative hypothalamic function in CP patients (Qi et al. 2012). Vimentin was found to be weak or negative in slightly over 40 % of ACPs and in 100 % of PCPs. When present, it was predominantly expressed in the peripheral, palisading cells. The stellate cells were consistently negative. Interestingly, vimentin was strongly expressed in the epithelial cells constituting the finger-like projections. About 38 % of ACP did not show any E-cadherin, whereas this adhesion molecule was constantly expressed in PCPs without differences between the centre and periphery of papillae. The authors showed a decrease in E-cadherin and increase in vimentin in ACPs that recurred against those that behaved more indolently.

2.5.1 Invasion in Craniopharyngioma and Its Implications

The issue of local invasion in CPs has been the object of much debate, and it therefore deserves a separate paragraph. CPs usually appear grossly well-circumscribed, but their microscopic margins are often irregular and intimately interconnected with the adjacent brain tissue. In fact, nearly all studies that examined the pathological features of CP describe 'fingers' or 'islands' of tumour tissue invading the adjacent normal tissue looking like tongues of tumour cells projecting into the parenchyma that can still be in continuity with the tumour bulk or appear as isolated, detached tumour nests. Despite its relevance, only a small number of studies have focussed on the transition zone between CP and surrounding normal structures such as hypothalamus, pituitary gland, pituitary stalk, basal ganglia, optic tract and brainstem (Adamson et al. 1990; Weiner et al. 1994; Kasai et al. 1997; Inenaga et al. 2004; Karavitaki et al. 2005; Kawamata et al. 2005). Of note that brain invasion is considerably more common in ACP than PCP and virtually absent in mixed tumours. In addition, invasion is more frequent in paediatric than adult ACPs (reviewed in Müller 2014). Kawamata et al. (2005) have recently attempted a classification of the tumour/brain interface that could help in predicting surgical removal and outcome. They analysed the boundary between tumour and adjacent brain in 15 cases of ACP and classified the features in three types. Type 1 is characterised by capsule-like tissue composed of tumour and chronic inflammation and facing a gliotic brain tissue. The plain of cleavage in type 1 cases is not well demarcated. Type 2 shows a clear cleavage between tumour and brain, whilst type 3 is characterised by interdigitations of neoplastic tissue into the adjacent hypothalamus or pituitary gland. The three types were equally distributed.

Brain tissue reacts to invasion with piloid gliosis that contains Rosenthal's fibres (Fig. 2.5). Specimens from the immediate periphery of ACP can almost entirely consist of Rosenthal fibre-rich gliotic tissue mimicking pilocytic astrocytoma. Differential diagnosis between pilocytic astrocytoma and ACP can be challenging on intraoperative frozen sections, particularly difficult in children and when ACPs are cystic. Rare ACP can also invade the skull base (Chen et al. 2013) (Fig. 2.5).

The question if microscopic brain invasion has an impact on tumour recurrence remains open. Some investigators have regarded reactive gliosis surrounding these foci of brain invasion as the major obstacle to total surgical removal, whilst others suggested that gliotic tissue could represent a margin of safety at the tumour/hypothalamus interface that could be exploited as surgical plane to achieve complete resection (reviewed in Weiner et al. 1994). Weiner et al. (1994) observed that when gross, totally removed microscopic foci of invasion did not seem to be predictive of

Fig. 2.5 Adamantinous craniopharyngioma is often invasive. Invasion can occur as digitiform projections of neoplastic tissue extending in the adjacent hypothalamus but still in continuity with the main lesion (**a**, HE – ×10) or as isolated, microscopic nests detached from the tumour bulk (**b**, HE – ×20); invasion elicits florid reactive gliosis with formation of Rosenthal's fibres mimicking pilocytic astrocytoma (**a** and **b**). Invasion of the sellar bone can also occur (**c**, HE – ×4)

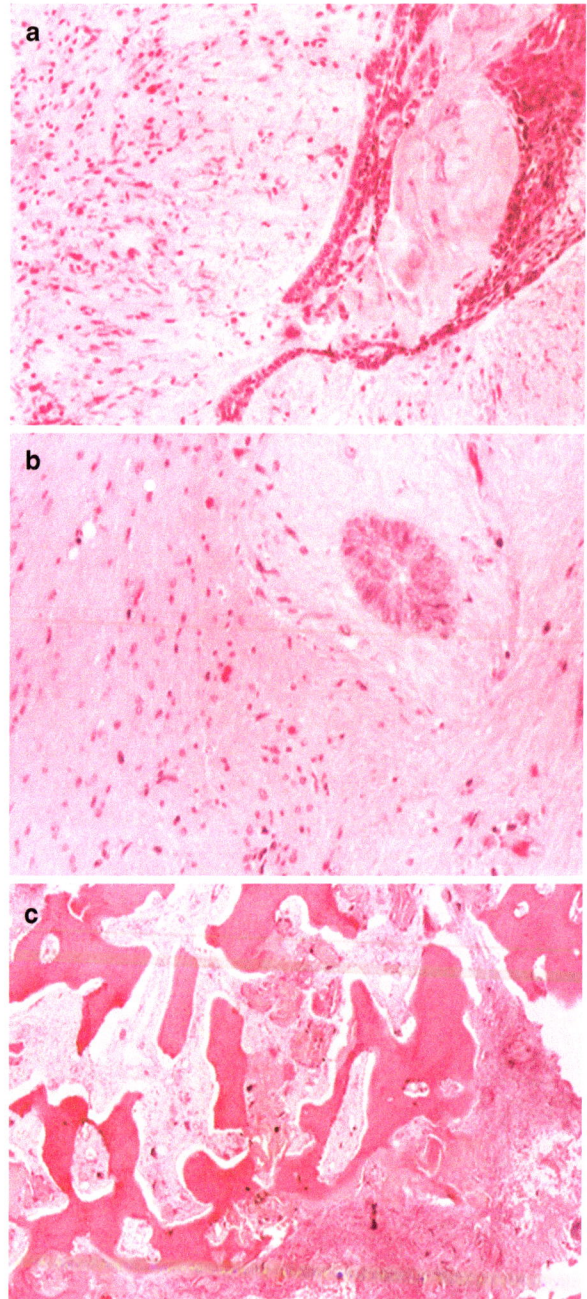

a higher rate of recurrence and suggested that invasion may merely represent inter-digitations of the tumour with the surrounding parenchyma.

Burghaus and co-authors (2010) investigated the brain invasion interface and showed that the tumours generate a specific cellular microenvironment. Using immunohistochemistry on tumour biopsies, they characterised the cellular environment of APC and compared the features with PCP. They observed a peculiar niche around the invasive edge of APC containing a population of cells with ramifying cytoplasmic processes and small nucleus that co-expressed nestin, GFAP and both the embryonic and the adult microtubule-associated protein 2 (MAP2). Overall, these features suggest that MAP2-positive cells could be glial progenitors rather than reactive astrocytes. Brain parenchyma at the interface also showed high tenas-cin-C expression. Similar features though less prominent were also seen in the brain tissue adjacent to some PCPs.

Other molecules that have positively been associated with outcome and found at the tumour/brain interface include cathepsins (Lubansu et al. 2003), retinoic acid and its receptors (Lefranc et al. 2003), osteonectin (Ebrahimi et al. 2013) and clau-din-1 (Stache et al. 2014).

Interested in the interplay between adhesion molecules at the boundary between CP and the adjacent structures, Lefranc and colleagues (2005) were the first to investigate systematically the pattern of integrins and galectins in CP cells as opposed to optic chiasm and infundibulum and their possible role in the formation of tumour projections that cause CPs to adhere to the surrounding tissue. The cohort study consisted of 50 ACPs, 19 of which occurred to children younger than 15 and 31 older adolescents and adults. Overall, the authors found that unlike optic chiasm and pituitary stalk, the expression of integrins and galectins in ACPs was heteroge-neous. The combined results of transcript analysis and immunohistochemistry dem-onstrated that ACPs express the α2, α6, αv, β1, β5 and β8 integrin subunits, whilst the optic chiasm and pituitary stalks express vitronectin, thrombospondin and col-lagens. α2, β1 and β8 integrin were widely distributed, whilst αv was low. When looking at other molecules of the extracellular matrix, they found that thrombospon-din, tenascin and collagen III were most frequently expressed in the optic chiasm and pituitary stalk, whereas vitronectin was only intensely expressed in the chiasm. The results suggested that APCs could adhere to the optic chiasm mainly via the interaction between α2/β1 and collagen, αv/β1 and vitronectin and αv/β5 and vitro-nectin and to the stalk via the interaction α2/β1 and collagen. Unlike the normal gland, Lefranc et al. observed no laminin and fibronectin in pituitary stalk but found thrombospondin and tenascin in both infundibulum and chiams, which are both ligands of integrins.

The members of the family of endogenous lectins 'galectins' can target integrin glycans and lead to their functional modulation. For this reason and once defined the pattern of integrins, the same authors went on investigating several galectins in their series of ACPs and found high and widespread expression of galectin-1 in most of the cases, whilst others showed patchy positivity with clusters of neoplastic cells displaying lower protein content. Galectin-3 was more extensively positive than galectin-1, but still some degree of variability was present. Galectin-4 was homogeneously weak and heterogeneous. The pattern of galectin-8 resembled and galectin-7 resembled galectin-3. Galectin-3 and galectin-7 featured the most intense immunolabelling. They also found that rapidly recurring tumours showed lower galectin-3 levels and that galectin-4 differed between gross total and incompletely resected ACPs, suggesting that galectin-4 could modulate the adhesion of tumour cells. Galectin-8 was variably expressed with a pattern similar to galectin-4, but it did not seem to be an independent predictor of recurrent likely because its preferred ligand α3-integrin was absent.

More recently, a series of Rathke's clef cysts (RCC), ACPs and PCPs were explored for the expression of claudin-1 (Stache et al. 2014). Membranous claudin-1 was documented in the basal layer of RCCs. Similar membranous but widespread expression was present in PAPs, whilst a strikingly lower expression was observed in ACPs, and when positive the protein appeared more cytoplasmic than on the plasma membrane. Whirl-like cell clusters in ACP that showed nuclear translocation of ß-catenin consistently lacked claudin-1.

The study of the mechanism causing brain invasion is however challenging on surgical specimens as they are often disrupted and include little brain tissue. In order to circumvent this problem and explore the molecular mechanism of invasion, Stache and colleagues have proposed a reproducible xenograft model of human ACP using the NMRI-Fox1nu/Fox1nu mutant mouse model (Stache et al. 2015). The model allowed the authors to explore tumour growth in its entirety and extend their studies to the invasive front into the adjacent brain. They implanted the tissue of three patients with ACP and conducted cell culture experiments and immunohistochemistry with samples from the same primary ACP. Engraftments were successful irrespective of the β-catenin status and age of the donor patient. Their model had also the advantages to allow the reconstruction of the whole tumour and characterise the cells initiating invasion. Tumour grafts replicated closely human ACPs including microcysts, calcifications and wet keratin. They showed the typical bordering zone between tumour and with piloid gliosis and the presence of undifferentiated neuroepithelial cells. Nine xenografts showed distinct invasion with the characteristic protrusions of tumour cells within the surrounding brain. The experiments documented the progression from a well-demarcated tumour with an intact basal cell layer to the invasive phase with initial formation of digitiform protrusions still retaining an intact basal cell layer and subsequent loss of outer cells and appearance of whirl-like neoplastic cells into the central nervous tissue. At this stage the outgrowing cells appear in direct contact with the extracellular matrix. Finally, the bordering cell layer seems to regenerate and wrap these clusters. Human ACP and xenografts were characterised for cytokeratin expression and cell proliferation. MIB-1 was negative in the whirl-like clusters, and the basal cell layer showed less cytokeratin, whilst there was nuclear β-catenin accumulation. Cells with nuclear β-catenin featured cytoplasmic and nuclear rather than membranous phosphorylated EGFR. Cell clusters were surrounded by claudin-1-expressing cells unlike the rest of the lesion that was claudin-1 negative.

2.6   Ectopic Locations

Craniopharyngiomas may recur after surgery in sites distant from the primary tumour. Such recurrence can be due to seeding along the surgical tract or seeding in the cerebrospinal fluid. In contrast, true ectopic examples in the absence of a sellar CP are rare. Defined as lesions that occur without any previous surgery and away from remnants of the Rathke's pouch, ectopic CPs have been documented in the cerebellopontine angle (Gökalp and Mertol 1990; Aquilina et al. 2006; Powers et al. 2007; Yan et al. 2009; Bozbuga et al. 2011; Kim et al. 2014), extracranially infrasellar without dural covering, clival (Kawamata et al. 2002) and petroclival region (Lee et al. 2009), ethmoid sinus (Jiang et al. 1998), fourth (Shah et al. 2007) ventricle, pineal gland (Solarski et al. 1978) and temporal (Banczerowski et al. 2007) and frontal lobes (Ortega-Porcayo et al. 2015). Their pathogenesis is unclear. A few cases occurred in patients with Gardner's syndrome (Aquilina et al. 2006; Bozbuga et al. 2011). Ectopic CPs are morphologically indistinguishable from their sellar and suprasellar counterparts. Their genetic makeup has not been fully investigated, and no previous studies have tested mutations of *CTNNB1* or BRAFV600E.

2.7   Metastatic Craniopharyngioma

Genuine metastatic CPs are rare but well documented, and unlike ectopic CPs, they occur in the presence of a sellar/suprasellar primary lesion. They can occur after long time after the operation of the primary tumour with one case described 21 years after surgery (Malik et al. 1992). Such remote recurrences can be secondary to implants of tumour fragments along the surgical path or due to dissemination and seeding in the subarachnoid space (reviewed in Frangou et al. 2009). The entire craniospinal axis can be involved including the cerebral hemispheres (Gupta et al. 1999; Ito et al. 2001; Elmaci et al. 2002; Bikmaz et al. 2009), posterior fossa (Bikmaz et al. 2009), lumbar spine (Lee et al. 2001), brainstem and basal ganglia (Novegno et al. 2002). Rare examples of epidural metastasis and patients with bilateral deposits have also been reported (reviewed in Frangou et al. 2009). It is unclear whether surgical manipulation contributes to dissemination, but it is worth noting that all reported metastases occurred in patients with suprasellar CP treated with transcranial approach but have never been documented in patients with an intrasellar lesion approached transsphenoidally. Both ACP and PCP were found to disseminate, but metastatic ACPs seem more common. Both children and adults can be affected. Interestingly, no distant deposits outside the CNS have ever been documented. Histologically, all cases of metastatic CP were similar to the primary tumour and showed no features of malignancy. Proliferation measured with Ki-67 is also not necessarily increased in CP that disseminated and their corresponding metastatic deposits. Some studies of Nishi et al. (1999) and Raghavan et al. (2000) documented higher mean indices than other authors in both primary and metastatic lesions, but others did not confirm this observation. Elmaci and colleagues (2002) used CD34 to examine the MVD of their case of PCP and its left temporoparietal metastasis and also looked VEGF expression and VEGFR2 mRNA identified by in situ hybridisation. They observed similar MVD in the primary tumour and metastasis but higher than the known MVD in nonrecurring CPs. VEGF expression was limited to connective tissue cells surrounding blood vessels in the primary tumour but was found in neoplastic cells in the metastatic deposit. Similarly, VEGFR2 transcripts were found exclusively in the capillary endothelium and pericytes in the primary CP but in both vessels and tumour cells of the metastasis deposit. Though the authors did not exclude the possibility of an artefact, this evidence led to the suggestion of a neoangiogenetic potential of CP cells that favour metastatic seeding.

2.8   Malignancy in Craniopharyngioma

CP can rarely present as a malignant lesion. Malignant transformation often results from progression of a benign CP with only occasional examples of malignant CP (mCP) occurring de novo (Rodriguez et al. 2007; Lauriola et al. 2011). Interestingly malignant transformation has almost exclusively been documented in ACP (mACP). One example of malignant PCP resulting from progression of a benign CP has been reported by Aquilina et al. (2010) in a 4-year-old boy who received radiotherapy after the initial operation.

To our knowledge, less than 30 cases of mCP have been documented since the original description in 1987 (Nelson et al. 1988; Akachi et al. 1987; Virik et al. 1999; Kristopaitis et al. 2000; Boongird et al. 2009; Gao et al. 2011; Lauriola et al. 2011; Wang et al. 2015).

Sofela and colleagues carried out an extensive literature search excluding studies reporting recurrent benign tumours with no histological evidence of malignancy and studies documenting metastatic but histologically benign CP. In addition to their 8-year-old patient, they reviewed 22 other patients (Sofela et al. 2014). The single case report by Salyer and Carter (1973) included by Sofela and colleagues likely represents a squamous cell carcinoma in epidermoid cyst rather than an example of mCP.

Malignant CP does not show any gender predilection with a male-to-female ratio of 9:10 and is more common in adults. Time between the initial diagnosis of ACP and the evidence of malignant transformation is broad and ranges from 3 to 55 years (median, 8.5 years). The median overall survival from the identification of malignant changes was only 6 months (range, 2 weeks–5 years). *De novo* mACP showed worse outcome with an overall survival of only 15 months from onset. mACP does not show any distinguishing features at preoperative neuroimaging, and similar to benign ACP, symptoms at onset include headaches, seizures and visual disorders.

Several patients underwent radiation therapy prior to developing an mCP. Paediatric mCPs, for instance, have only been documented in patients previously treated with radiotherapy leading to the suggestion that mCP could be radio induced. Unlike previously suggested, Sofela and co-authors (2014) found little evidence supporting the radiation-induced malignant transformation.

The diagnosis of mACP is essentially based on histological features, although no morphological criteria have been defined. General features of malignancy including cellular atypia, nuclear hyperchromasia and pleomorphism, high mitotic count, atypical mitoses and necrosis reminiscent of otherwise conventional squamous cell carcinoma and infiltration of surrounding structures are diagnostic features (Fig. 2.6). Not all reported cases contained areas of conventional ACP, though focal wet keratin and calcification are always seen. The malignant component usually shows features of squamous cell carcinoma; ameloblastic, columnar, odontogenic and myoepithelial cell carcinomas occurred less commonly. Extensive microvascular proliferation, prominent inflammation and reactive gliosis of the adjacent brain parenchyma are common. One case (Rodriguez et al. 2007) demonstrated myoepitheliomatous elements expressing smooth muscle actin and p63, giving a remarkable resemblance to a salivary gland myoepithelial neoplasm. Histological features of two cases (Kristopaitis et al. 2000; Rodriguez et al. 2007) resembled odontogenic ghost cell carcinoma.

Similar to benign ACP, malignant examples showed nuclear immunostaining for ß-catenin. Intense nuclear labelling for p53, variable expression of p16 and usually high MIB-1 labelling index have also been reported (Rodriguez et al. 2007). VEGF expression was examined in some cases but found similar in the malignant and benign components, but MVD appeared considerably higher in the malignant areas than the conventional ACP component.

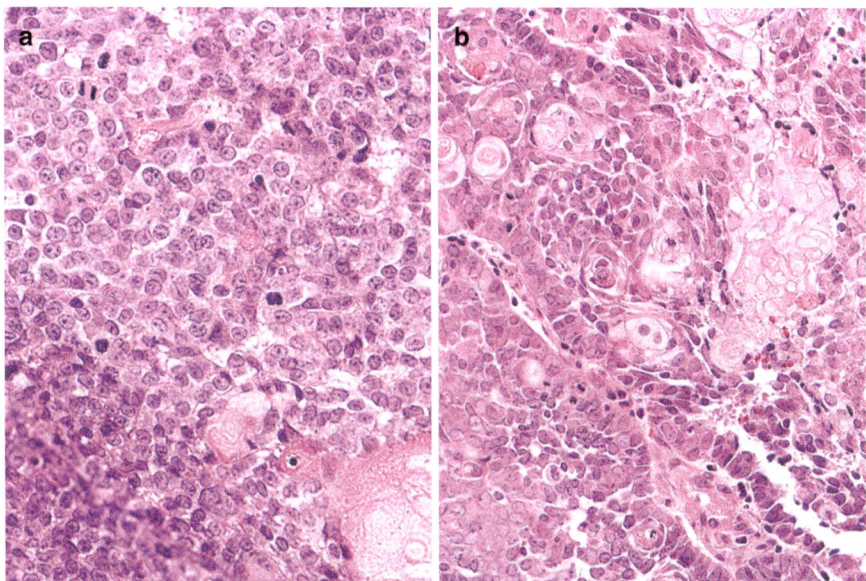

Fig. 2.6 Malignant craniopharyngioma can be present de novo as undifferentiated epithelial tumour (**a**, HE – ×20) or result from the progression of a benign craniopharyngioma (**b**, HE – ×20). Cellular atypia and brisk mitotic activity are the hallmarks of malignant examples (Courtesy of Dr. Fausto Rodriguez, Division of Neuropathology, John Hopkins University, Boston MA, USA)

Multiple recurrences of benign ACP before malignant transformation are the norm. Brain invasion is a common feature of mCP, making resection and radiotherapy planning very difficult. Prognosis is dismal with a mean overall survival of 4 months. Only one patient (Kristopaitis et al. 2000) survived longer than 5 years after the occurrence of malignant transformation. Distant metastases have however never been reported. Given the rarity of mCP, there is currently no general consensus for the management of patients.

2.9   Differential Diagnosis: Lesions Mimicking Craniopharyngioma

Cystic lesions of the sella turcica and suprasellar region encompass histologically defined clinicopathological entities including RCC, epidermoid cysts, dermoid cysts and CP with RCC and CP sitting at the opposite ends of the spectrum (Harrison et al. 1994).

However, a significant overlap exists reflecting the suggested common embryological derivation of these lesions from ectodermal cell remnants of Rathke's pouch and the craniopharyngeal duct. It is known that neuroimaging features may be similar and that distinction between different cystic lesions of the sellar and suprasellar region can also be difficult at histological examination particularly when only biopsies are available (Harrison et al. 1994; Zada et al. 2010; Ren et al. 2012).

In several cysts, the epithelial lining may show indeterminate and nonspecific features, making the categorisation of the lesion challenging (Shin et al. 1999). Harrison et al. (1994) recognised overlapping features in between epidermoid and dermoid cysts and CP consisting of extensive regions where the keratohyalin granule layer was absent from squamous epithelium. Squamous metaplasia in RCC epithelium is also a cause of confusion. In addition, RCC with squamous metaplasia may contain dense, 'motor oil' fluid similar to that commonly seen in ACP.

To stress the difficulties in distinguishing between cystic sellar lesions, Crotty and colleagues (1995) reported two illustrative cases that represent pitfalls in the diagnosis of PCP. The first patient in particular, a 22-year-old man, presented with a 2-year history of impaired vision, and headache was diagnosed with RCC with squamous metaplasia on the initial biopsy. Similar diagnosis was made on the recurrent lesion, 3 months after the first biopsy. The second recurrence 4 months thereafter conversely showed typical PCP. The importance of correlating neuroimaging and surgical findings with the histology cannot be stressed enough in challenging cases.

Mixed lesions with otherwise typical features of ACP or PCP but also displaying columnar, focally ciliated epithelium in keeping with RCC have been documented, raising the suggestion that some CP may develop from pre-existent RCC (Fig. 2.7) (Oka et al. 1997; Okada et al. 2010; Alomari et al. 2015).

Evidence of nuclear immunostain for β-catenin (Hofmann et al. 2006) in squamous epithelium and the recent discovery of BRAFV600E mutations in over 90 % PCP (see paragraph on molecular aspects) and the development on an antibody directed against the mutant BRAF protein have partly resolved the issue of differentiating between RCC with squamous metaplasia and PCP (Schweizer et al. 2014;

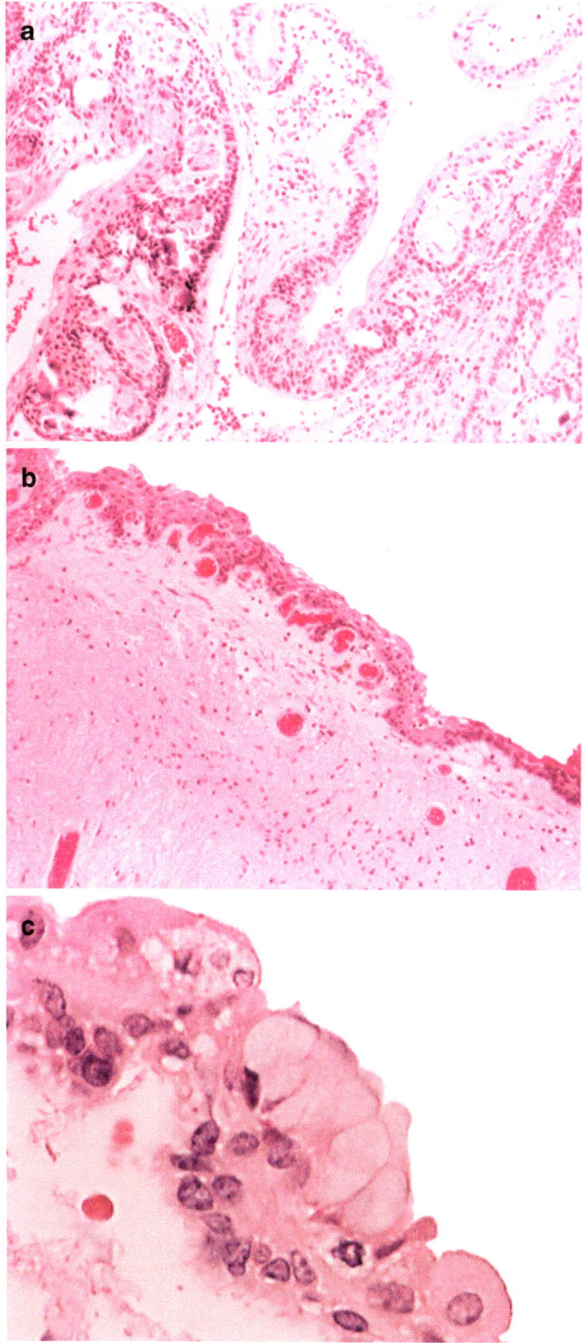

Fig. 2.7 Craniopharyngiomas can at times contain areas reminiscent of a Rathke's cleft cyst. The cyst wall of this adamantinous craniopharyngioma (**a**, HE – ×4) focally shows pluristratified squamous epithelium (**b**, HE – ×10) with goblet cells (**c**, HE – ×40)

Kim et al. 2015). The antibody currently used for the detection of mutant protein may give weak immunolabelling (Schweizer et al. 2015) and also nonspecific staining due to a cross reaction with axonemal dyneins (Jones et al. 2015). Several authors investigated the pattern of cytokeratin expression in CP and RCC. Xin et al. suggested that cytokeratins 8 and 20 are preferentially expressed in RCC irrespective of the presence of squamous metaplasia but are negative in ACP and PCP (Xin et al. 2002). Le and colleagues (2007) could not confirm these findings.

To further complicate the field, sellar tumours with 'transitional' features including elements of RCC, squamous epithelium and pituitary adenoma have respectively been described by Kepes (1978) and Nishio and colleagues (1987).

The distinction between a CP and epidermoid cyst may be difficult and at times impossible on conventional HE-stained sections and even using immunohistochemistry. For instance, Netsky (1988) found that fully one-third of the cases displayed a transitional histology between that of an epidermoid cyst and a CP.

Xanthogranuloma (XG) of the sellar region represents another lesion that enters the differential diagnosis with ACP. Sellar XG is composed of cholesterol clefts, macrophages, chronic inflammatory cellular reaction and hemosiderin deposits that can mimic CP at histological examination (Fig. 2.8). Paulus et al. (1999) reviewed 110 cases originally diagnosed as CP and identified 37 lesions with distinct xanthogranulomatous features. Age, site and outcome of the 37 patients differed from CP. Sellar XG occurs predominantly in adolescents and young adults. When compared with CP, XG appears to have smaller size, longer preoperative history, lower frequency of visual impairment, better resectability and an overall more favourable outcome. XG in children shows high rates of hypothalamic involvement and intra- and extrasellar localisation (92 %) and a comparable rate of endocrine deficiencies when compared with CP.

Distinction between sellar and suprasellar cystic lesion has prognostic relevant implications, and an erroneous diagnosis can lead to inadequate treatment. In fact,

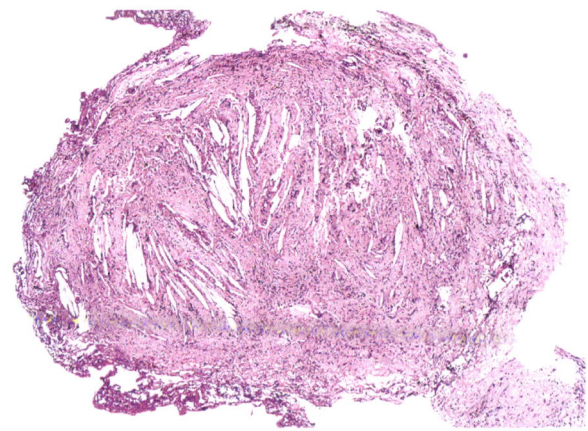

Fig. 2.8 Whole mount of a case of sellar xanthogranuloma; note the abundance of cholesterol clefts mimicking craniopharyngioma

outcome of RCC, epidermoid and dermoid cysts and XG is more favourable than CP, and these lesions do not require radiotherapy (Mukherjee et al. 1997). Upon review of children enrolled in HIT-Endo and KRANIOPHARYNGEOM 2000, Müller and colleagues (2010) compared the outcomes of 117 patients with CP against 14 children with RCC and 14 with XG. 5-year progression-free survival for RCC was 85 %, but children showed considerable endocrine morbidity. The outcome in XG was favourable, showing no relapse or progression after surgical treatment. Furthermore, hypothalamic obesity at initial presentation or as sequelae was not a clinical feature in XG, despite the considerable high rate of anterior hypothalamic involvement.

Han et al. (2014) have recently conducted a detailed literature review of RCC including natural history and post-surgical outcomes. They found great variability of recurrence rates among studies from 0 % to up to 42 % with a more reassuring 16–18 % recurrence rate at 5 years in the largest series. RCC in children and adolescents has smaller intrasellar size and does not show hypothalamic involvement, therefore causing pituitary deficiencies without post-surgical hypothalamic sequelae. Interestingly inflammation and reactive squamous metaplasia in the cyst wall are associated with higher recurrence rate than cyst lined by mucinous, ciliated cells (13–31 % recurrence rates), further raising concerns in the differential diagnosis between RCC and CP.

2.10 Craniopharyngioma Can Occur in Association with Other Sellar Lesions

Craniopharyngioma can occur in association with other sellar lesions including pituitary adenoma (reviewed in Jin et al. 2013; Finzi et al. 2014), germ cell tumours (Barbounis et al. 2013) fatsdand sellar chordoma (Belza 1966). Pituitary adenoma accounts for the commonest associated lesion, and lactotroph adenoma is the most frequent type (Wheatley et al. 1986; Asari et al. 1987; Cusimano et al. 1988; Guaraldi et al. 2013) possibly reflecting the high incidence of sporadic prolactinomas in the general population. All the other types of adenoma have been documented including gonadotroph adenoma (Karavitaki et al. 2008; Sargis et al. 2009), somatotropinoma (Prabhakar et al. 1971), ACTH (Finzi et al. 2014), thyrotroph (Yoshida et al. 2008) and silent type III (Moshkin et al. 2009) adenomas. Adenoma and CP can be distinct, therefore appearing as a collision tumour, but also and more interestingly, the two components can be admixed with islands of palisading epithelium around loose stroma with stellate cells typical of CP being as haphazardly distributed within the adenoma (Yoshida et al. 2008; Gokden and Mrak 2009; Finzi et al. 2014). The CP component in the cases documented so far accounted for a variable proportion of the overall neoplastic population ranging from 5 to 40 % and had adamantinous features. A transition between ACP and adenoma has been described in some examples suggesting a common origin of the endocrine and squamous components. For instance, the ACP component in the case published by Yoshida and colleagues in a gonadotropinoma expressed the steroidogenic factor 1 that is a nuclear transcription factor for the gonadotroph lineage (Yoshida et al. 2008). More recently, Finzi et al. (2014) reported on a mixed ACP and silent ACTH macroadenoma in a 75-year-old woman presented with diplopia due to a sixth left nerve palsy. The ACP component was multiple foci of transition between CP and adenoma. ACP cells did not show any neuroendocrine markers or hormones, but rare adenomatous cells showed nuclear p40 immunoreactivity suggesting a divergent differentiation from the CP (Fig. 2.9). The adenoma cells showed intense and complete membranous immunoreactivity for β-catenin, whilst expression was weaker and often incomplete in ACP cells. 'Hybrid' tumour cells with features of both ACP and pituitary adenoma were then observed ultrastructurally where small dense neurosecretory granules coexisted with bundles of cytoplasmic filaments and desmosomes indicating mixed endocrine and squamous differentiation. The authors suggested a possible origin of such mixed forms from multipotent stem/progenitor cells in the adult pituitary.

Two children with Cushing's syndrome and ACP but without histological evidence of corticotroph adenoma or ACTH expression in CP cells have also been reported. Hypercortisolemia resolved postoperatively in both patients indicating that that was somehow related to ACP, but the cause of Cushing's syndrome remained unresolved (Ackland et al. 1987; Caceres et al. 2005).

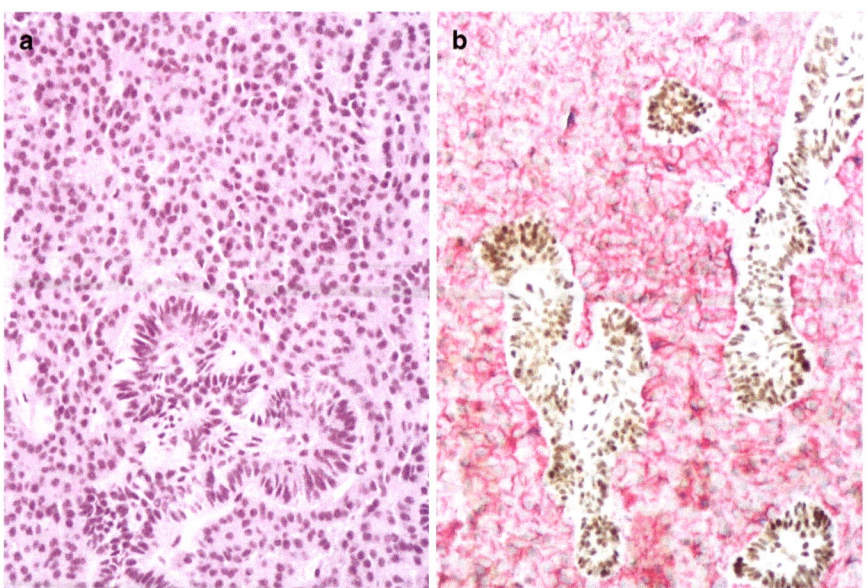

Fig. 2.9 Mixed pituitary adenoma and adamantinous craniopharyngioma; islands of squamous epithelium with palisading features are admixed with neuroendocrine cells of the pituitary adenoma (**a** – HE, ×20); double immunohistochemistry shows that adenoma cells express chromogranin A, a marker of endocrine differentiation, whilst craniopharyngioma cells are positive for p40, a marker of squamous differentiation (**b** – ABC peroxidase – ×20; *red* chromogranin A, *brown* p40) (Courtesy Dr. Stefano La Rosa, University of Insubria, Varese, Italy)

2.11 Molecular Aspects and Pathogenesis

The understanding of the molecular mechanisms underlying the pathogenesis of CP has progressed considerably in the last few years with the discovery of mutations in the gene encoding β-catenin in ACP and the mutation of BRAFV600E in PCP. Before such progress, genetic studies looking at chromosomal abnormalities produced discrepant results. In fact, multiple translocations and deletions were reported in a limited number of paediatric ACPs using classic cytogenetic analysis (Gorski et al. 1992; Karnes et al. 1992), whilst no aberrations were found by others (Griffin et al. 1992; Bhattacharjee et al. 1997). Studies with CGH showed similar conflicting results. Reinstein and colleagues found aberrations in six of their nine adult and paediatric ACPs including Yp loss in one case and multiple gains in the remaining lesions (Rienstein et al. 2003), whilst two large studies overall investigating 39 cases of ACP and PCP in adult and children failed to show significant chromosomal imbalances (Rickert and Paulus 2003; Yoshimoto et al. 2004).

Such contradictory results even obtained in homogeneous series suggest that chromosomal aberrations do not play a role in the pathogenesis of CP.

Studying X chromosome inactivation analysis, it has been demonstrated that at least a subset of CPs is monoclonal in origin (Sarubi et al. 2001), therefore suggesting that an acquired somatic mutation could have been responsible for the pathogenesis of CP (reviewed in Hussain et al. 2013). Unlike several other types of cancer, mutations in the gene encoding the tumour suppressor protein *P53* were found to be uncommon in CP (reviewed in Prieto et al. 2013). The transcription factor *CDX2* has not been documented in any of the ACP or PCP investigated (Schittenhelm et al. 2010). Likewise, CPs do not harbour any mutations in transcription factor genes *HESX1*, *PROP1* and *POU1F12* (Campanini et al. 2010). Campanini and colleagues also looked at miRNA and noted a deregulation of miRNAs CP, leading to the suggestion of their potential involvement in the pathogenesis and modulation of the Wnt signalling (Campanini et al. 2010). Mutations in the tumour suppressor gene *PTCH* that is responsible for Gorlin's syndrome are uncommon (Sarubi et al. 2001; Musani et al. 2006).

It is worth noting that several cytogenetics and CGH studies had the limitation of not distinguishing between childhood and adult CP. The heterogeneity of results may therefore reflect the heterogeneity of disease. In addition, some of the published studies have analysed CPs that were previously treated with radiotherapy, therefore identifying random and nonrandom abnormalities that were treatment induced rather than typical of CP.

2.11.1 Molecular Aetiology of Adamantinous Craniopharyngioma

In recent years it has become established that over-activation of the WNT/β–catenin signalling pathway underlies the molecular aetiology of human ACP. This pathway plays a critical role during embryonic development as well as in adulthood and when dysregulated can cause disease, including cancer. The activation of the WNT/β–catenin is tightly regulated by levels of stabilised β-catenin in the cytoplasm. In the absence of WNT ligands, β-catenin is trapped in a cytoplasmic 'destruction' complex formed by several proteins including the scaffold proteins adenomatous polyposis coli (APC) and axin and the protein kinases GSK3β and CKIα. Through this complex, β-catenin is phosphorylated by GSK3β and CKIα in specific regulatory amino acids located in its N-terminus, and this posttranslational mark is recognised by ubiquitin, activating the ubiquitin–proteasome pathway resulting in β-catenin degradation. Binding of WNT ligands to the membrane-located Frizzled receptors leads to disassembly of the destruction complex, causing β-catenin stabilisation due to impaired phosphorylation and degradation. As a consequence, β-catenin protein accumulates in the cytoplasm and translocates to the nucleus where it binds TCF/LEF transcription factors to activate transcription of direct targets, such as *Myc*, *Ccnd1*, *Axin2* and *Bmp4* (He et al. 1998; Tetsu and McCormick 1999; Jho et al. 2002; Kim et al. 2002).

Mutations in gene encoding β-catenin *CTNNB1* have been identified in most of the human ACP samples analysed (Buslei et al. 2005; Sekine et al. 2002; Kato et al. 2004; Oikonomou et al. 2005; Brastianos et al. 2014). These mutations result in the substitution or deletion of the critical regulatory N-terminal phosphorylation amino acids that control β-catenin stabilisation and are predicted to cause its nuclear–cytoplasmic accumulation and over-activation of the WNT/β–catenin pathway. In agreement with this prediction, nuclear–cytoplasmic accumulation of β-catenin is observed in most of human ACP tumours, usually in small groups of cells that form clusters (hereafter referred to as 'cell clusters') and in single cells throughout the tumours (Buslei et al. 2007) (Fig. 2.10). These clusters represent a histological hallmark of human ACP that distinguishes it from any other tumour of the sellar region, including PCP (Buslei et al. 2007; Hofmann et al. 2006). Of note, PCP has been shown to be associated with over-activating mutations in BRAF (Buslei et al. 2005; Larkin et al. 2014). As

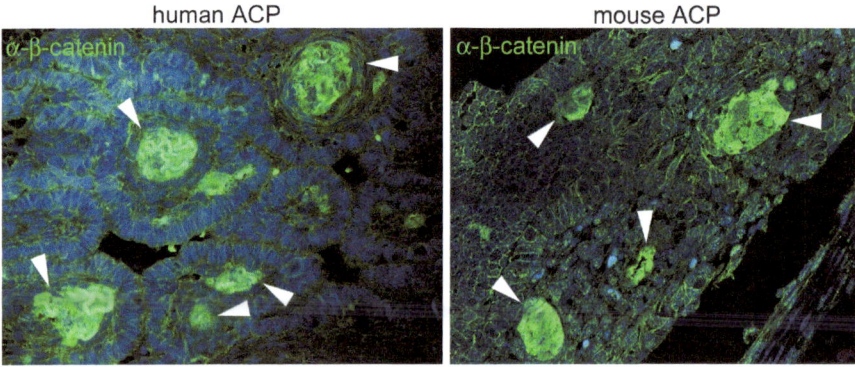

Fig. 2.10 Nuclear–cytoplasmic β-catenin accumulation occurs only in cell clusters in both human and mouse ACP. Immnunostaining against β-catenin on histological sections of human and mouse adamantinous craniopharyngioma (*arrowhead*). Most of the cells show membranous staining, and only small groups of cells, which forms clusters, accumulate nuclear–cytoplasmic β-catenin

expected, the activation of the WNT/β–catenin pathway is mostly restricted to the cluster cells as revealed by the expression of the transcriptional targets *AXIN2*, *LEF1* and *BMP4* (Holsken et al. 2009; Sekine et al. 2004; Gaston-Massuet et al. 2011). Using a novel xenotransplant model for human ACP, the activity of the clusters has been shown to be important for controlling the infiltrative behaviour into the brain (Stache et al. 2014). These cluster cells express some markers associated with stemness and are not proliferative (Holsken et al. 2014). These initial human studies clearly provided enough evidence for a role of *CTNNB1* mutations and the WNT pathway in the aetiology of ACP. However, whether these mutations are driving tumorigenesis could not be concluded from these experiments.

The generation of genetically engineered mouse models is a powerful approach to assess the role of specific genetic aberrations in the aetiology of human cancers because it allows the expression of potentially oncogenic mutations in the specific tissues from where neoplasms derive. An initial mouse model for human ACP was generated by expressing in Rathke's pouch (RP) a degradation-resistant mutant form of β-catenin that causes the over-activation of the WNT/β–catenin pathway, similar to the commonly identified human mutations. The RP is the embryonic primordium of the anterior pituitary and is derived from the oral ectoderm. It contains the progenitors that give rise to all of the cell types of the mature anterior pituitary (i.e. somatotrophs, lactotrophs, thyrotrophs, corticotrophs, gonadotrophs and melanotrophs) as well as the Sox2+ve pituitary stem cells (Andoniadou et al. 2007; Davis et al. 2011; Jayakody et al. 2012). Therefore, in this ACP mouse model, a mutant form of β-catenin functionally equivalent to that identified in human ACP was expressed in the embryonic epithelial cells, from where human ACP is thought to derive (i.e. the remnants of RP).

These mice develop pituitary tumours, which upon histological and molecular examination were similar to human ACP (Gaston-Massuet et al. 2011). For instance, murine tumours showed β-catenin-accumulating cell clusters with concomitant expression of *Lef1*, *Axin2 and Bmp4*, indicating the activation of the WNT pathway (Andoniadou et al. 2012; Gaston-Massuet et al. 2011). These cell clusters displayed a whirl-like morphology and low to absent proliferation capacity as assessed by the lack of expression of Ki-67, a marker of cycling cells. In addition, they expressed other markers such as sonic hedgehog (*Shh*) and *Cxcr4*, which are also expressed in human clusters (Andoniadou et al. 2012; Gong et al. 2014). However, the mouse tumours did not show calcification or deposits of wet keratin, and so far, infiltration of the tumour into the hypothalamus has not been observed, suggesting that these characteristics may represent species-specific differences (e.g. human ACP is thought to develop in years, whilst mouse ACP develops in weeks). These experiments demonstrated a causative effect of mutant β-catenin in the initiation of ACP, thus confirming the hypotheses drawn from the human studies.

2.11.2 Stem Cells Play a Critical Role in ACP Tumorigenesis

To understand how tumours develop, it is important to identify not only driver mutations but also the cell types in which these genetic aberrations exert an oncogenic effect. The mouse model previously described represents an excellent tool to address which cells within the pituitary need to be targeted with oncogenic β-catenin for ACP to develop.

Using several murine transgenic lines, oncogenic β-catenin was expressed in terminally differentiated and committed precursors of both the embryonic and adult glands, but no tumours developed (Gaston-Massuet et al. 2011). These differentiated and committed cells are cycling and proliferative during development and early stages of postnatal life, therefore demonstrating that their resistance to tumorigenesis is not due to quiescence. These experiments demonstrated an essential role for undifferentiated embryonic precursors of RP in the genesis of ACP and fostered the hypothesis that other undifferentiated precursors or stem cells in the adult pituitary might also be capable of generating tumours.

The existence of stem cells in the adult pituitary gland has been controversial until recently due to the lack of in vivo evidence. In vitro, pituitary stem cells (PSCs) capable of self-renewing and differentiating into hormone-producing cells have been identified in the adult gland by several groups (Lepore et al. 2005; Gleiberman et al. 2008; Fauquier et al. 2008; Garcia-Lavandeira et al. 2009; de Almeida et al. 2010; Castinetti et al. 2011; Florio 2011; Vankelecom 2012). The in vitro assay used in these studies measures the potential of dissociated pituitary cells to clonally expand in culture either as adherent colonies or floating spheres. Although several markers have been associated with PSCs, the clonogenic potential of the adult pituitary resides in cells contained within the Sox2+ve and Sox9+ve populations, as demonstrated in in vitro assays using cells isolated by flow cytometry (Andoniadou et al. 2013; Rizzoti et al. 2013). In follow-up studies, genetic tracing was performed in vivo using genetically engineered mice expressing a tamoxifen-inducible form of the Cre recombinase in adult Sox2+ve or Sox9+ve cells. In these strains, the activation of Cre results in the expression of yellow fluorescence protein (YFP) in the Sox2+ve and Sox9+ve cells and their progeny, allowing the genetic tracing of these lineages. These experiments revealed that the Sox2+ve and Sox9+ve progeny populate all of the hormone-producing cells and contribute to normal cell turn over in the adult pituitary, thus demonstrating that they are stem cells in vivo. Of note, Sox2+ve and Sox9+ve cells are also present in human pituitaries, where they may play a similar role to their murine counterparts (Kelberman et al. 2008; Garcia-Lavandeira et al. 2009).

Tissue-specific adult stem cells can also be the cell of origin of tumours and cancers. The cancer stem cell (CSC) paradigm proposes that within the tumour mass, only restricted numbers of cells have the capacity to self-renew and give rise to differentiated tumour cells (Clarke and Fuller 2006; Alison et al. 2008; Nguyen et al. 2012; Visvader and Lindeman 2012). For instance, familial adenomatous polyposis (FAP) is an inherited disorder associated with inactivating mutations in APC resulting in over-activation of the WNT/β–catenin pathway. Patients with FAP often develop multiple tumours called adenomas (polyps), which can subsequently progress to colorectal cancer. In the mouse, the deletion of APC in the stem cells located at the base of the intestinal crypts generates tumours that resemble the polyps observed in human patients (Barker et al. 2009). Similarly, the over-activation of the

WNT pathway by expressing oncogenic β-catenin (the same mutant protein used in the mouse ACP models) also leads to the formation of multiple intestinal adenomas in mice (Zhu et al. 2009). Of relevance, genetic tracing of the mutated crypt stem cells in mice revealed that the polyps were YFP+ve, indicating that tumours are derived from the targeted stem cells. These experiments demonstrate that normal crypt stem cells can be mutated by oncogenic proteins to generate CSCs. As CSCs may be especially resistant to common cancer therapies (chemo- and radiotherapy), the implications of this model are important from a therapeutic perspective, as not only the bulk of the tumour cells should be eliminated but also the scarce population of CSCs must be targeted by anticancer treatments.

In the context of the CSC paradigm, it was important to determine whether Sox2+ve stem cells in the adult pituitary could be transformed into CSCs by expressing oncogenic mutant β-catenin. A *Sox2-CreERT2* mouse line was used to simultaneously express oncogenic β-catenin and YFP in Sox2+ve cells in the adult pituitary, which resulted in tumour formation (Andoniadou et al. 2012). These tumours were undifferentiated and did not express synaptophysin, a characteristic common with human ACP. Unexpectedly, however, the tumours were not YFP+ve, indicating that tumour cells were not the progeny of the mutated Sox2+ve stem cells. Further analyses revealed that Sox2+ve cells proliferated transiently and stop proliferating, giving rise to clusters with nuclear–cytoplasmic β-catenin accumulation that were similar to the typical clusters observed in human ACP.

If the tumours are not derived from the mutated Sox2+ve cells, how do tumours form? It was shown that cluster cells express a myriad of signalling molecules including SHH, members of the TGF-β, WNT and FGF families of secreted proteins as well as numerous chemokines and cytokines, which are all capable of influencing the tumour environment in an autocrine and/or paracrine manner (Andoniadou et al. 2012). This prompted the proposal of a paracrine model of involvement of tissue-specific stem cells in tumorigenesis that is conceptually different to the CSC paradigm, as the cell sustaining the oncogenic mutation and the cell of origin of the tumours are different (Fig. 2.11) (Andoniadou et al. 2013). Further research will reveal whether this model is applicable to other pituitary tumours and human cancers, but published evidence suggests broader implications of this model in the oncology field (Nicolas et al. 2003; Demehri et al. 2009; Lujambio et al. 2013; Kode et al. 2014; Caretti et al. 2014; Deschene et al. 2014).

In summary, research in human and mouse models supports the notion that mutations in β-catenin leading to the over-activation of the WNT pathway specifically in pituitary embryonic precursors or adult stem cells are necessary and sufficient to induce ACP.

2.11.3 The EGFR and SHH Pathways Are Upregulated in Mouse and Human ACP

Despite the critical role of over-activated WNT/β–catenin signalling in several human tumours and cancers, so far no specific pathway inhibitors with therapeutic

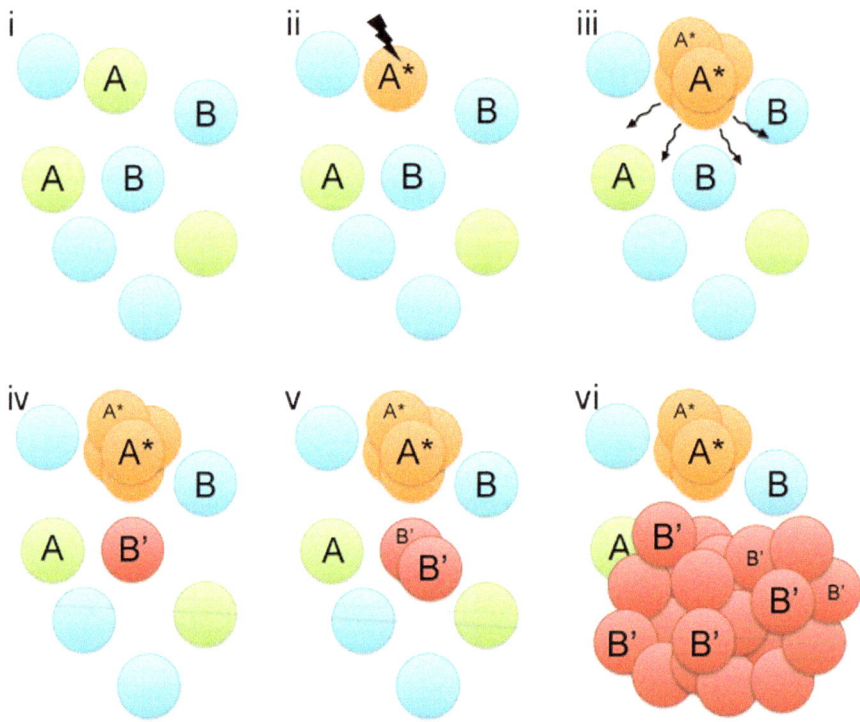

Fig. 2.11 Paracrine model for the involvement of pituitary stem cells in tumorigenesis; (**i**) schematic representation of Sox2+ve stem cells (*A*) and Sox2-ve cells in the adult pituitary. Expression of oncogenic β-catenin in some Sox2+ve cells (*A** in **ii**) results in transient proliferation and formation of β-catenin-accumulating cell clusters (*A** in **iii** and **iv**) and the release of secreted factors to the surrounding cells (**ii**) leading to cell transformation (*B′*), proliferation (*B′* in **v**) and tumour formation (*B′* in **vi**)

value have been identified. Therefore, there is a need for a better understanding of the genes and pathways that are deregulated in human ACP, if we aim to develop specific chemical treatments against these aggressive tumours. Two major pathways have been recently identified, which hold the promise of being easily targetable: the epithelial growth factor receptor (EGFR) and the sonic hedgehog (SHH) pathways.

EGFR is a cell surface receptor tyrosine kinase for the epidermal growth factor (EGF) family of extracellular ligands. Ligand binding (e.g. EGF) induces receptor dimerisation, intrinsic intracellular tyrosine kinase activation and subsequent autophosphorylation of multiple tyrosine residues (p-EGFR). This process initiates signal transduction through several intracellular cascades resulting in the regulation of cell proliferation, differentiation, apoptosis and motility (Mendelsohn and Baselga 2000; Herbst 2004). Over-activated EGFR signalling has been identified in several cancers such as non-small cell lung cancer, colorectal carcinoma, breast cancer, head and neck squamous carcinoma, bladder cancer and pancreatic cancer (Ono and

Kuwano 2006). The activation of the pathway can be caused by the increased expression of ligands and receptors, *EGFR* gene amplification and EGFR mutations leading to the constitutive activation of EGFR signalling (Laurent-Puig et al. 2009).

Recently, immunostaining with specific antibodies against p-EGFR revealed the activation of the pathway in human ACP, specifically within the β-catenin-accumulating cell clusters (Holsken et al. 2011). This is consistent with the increased expression of EGF in cell clusters in the ACP mouse model (Andoniadou et al. 2012), suggesting an autocrine signalling mechanism (Andoniadou et al. 2012). So far, genetic aberrations in the EGFR pathway have not been identified in human ACP, indicating that the over-activation of the pathway is ligand dependent (Holsken et al. 2009). A specific small-molecule compound known as gefitinib (Iressa™), which belongs to the group of low-molecular-weight anilinoquinazolines, is a highly specific EGFR inhibitor and approved as chemotherapeutic agent for the treatment of non-small cell lung cancer and currently tested against other solid tumours (Ono and Kuwano 2006; Herbst et al. 2004). Of note, gefitinib is able to inhibit cell motility of human ACP primary cultured cells (Holsken et al. 2009).

The hedgehog (HH) pathway is required during embryogenesis and plays an important role in stem cells (Ingham and Placzek 2006; Alvarez-Medina et al. 2009; Shin et al. 2011). HH secreted signals (e.g. SHH) bind to the receptor patched 1 (*PTCH1*) leading to the derepression of the transducer smoothened (*SMO*). Activated SMO initiates the intracellular signalling cascade that culminates in the nuclear translocation of GLI proteins, ultimately causing the transcriptional activation of target genes, including *GLI* and *PTCH1* (Ingham and Placzek 2006). Inactivating mutations in PTCH1 are commonly found in most sporadic medulloblastomas (Romer et al. 2004; Yauch et al. 2008; Gibson et al. 2010) and in Gorlin syndrome (also known as nevoid basal cell carcinoma syndrome), a rare condition in which patients have increased risk of developing medulloblastoma, rhabdomyosarcoma, basal cell carcinoma and occasionally craniopharyngioma (Theunissen and de Sauvage 2009; Musani et al. 2006). Other cancers, including leukaemia, small-cell lung cancer, breast cancer and pancreatic, prostate and gastrointestinal malignancies, also exhibit over-active HH pathway, but this is caused by increased expression of SHH ligand without known mutations in pathway components (Theunissen and de Sauvage 2009; Yauch et al. 2008).

Gene expression profiling of cluster versus non-cluster cells in ACP mouse models revealed the overexpression of SHH in the β-catenin-accumulating cell clusters (Andoniadou et al. 2012, 2013). This finding prompted the analysis of SHH expression in human ACP, which demonstrated the presence of *SHH* mRNA restricted to the β-catenin-accumulating cell clusters (Andoniadou et al. 2012). Moreover, expression of *PTCH1* was detected within and surrounding the cell clusters, suggesting that secreted SHH protein may be acting over a distance as a morphogen (Andoniadou et al. 2012). So far, mutations in components of the HH pathway have not been described in human ACP.

The demonstration that the SHH pathway is active in ACP may have important therapeutical implications. Several preclinical studies in mice have demonstrated the efficacy of SMO inhibitors in reducing tumour burden in mouse models for human cancers (Romer et al. 2004; Rubin and de Sauvage 2006; Bijlsma and Roelink 2010). In addition, SMO inhibitors were shown to have a transient but robust anticancer effect in a patient with metastatic medulloblastoma, suggesting that inhibition of the HH pathway might be potentially beneficial (Rudin et al. 2009). Currently, no information is available on the anti-tumoral effect of SMO inhibitors in human ACP.

2.11.4 Molecular Aetiology of Papillary Craniopharyngioma

The observation of mutations in exon 3 of *CTNNB1* encoding a degradation targeting motif of β-catenin has been a major contribution to the understanding of the pathogenesis of ACP.

Brastianos and colleagues (Brastianos et al. 2014) performed whole exome sequencing of 12 APC and 3 PCP and targeted genotyping of 95 additional cases. Because neoplastic tissue in CPs is often admixed with a large amount of reactive, inflammatory cells and stromal cells, the authors expected a contamination by normal cells and therefore analysed the results of sequencing with MuTect that is designed to identify somatic mutations with very low allelic fractions.

The two adult and the paediatric PCPs in the authors' discovery cohort harboured the clonal mutation c.1799T > A in the oncogene *BRAF*. Such mutation causing the substitution V600E is common in cancer and is known to constitutively activate this serine–threonine kinase that regulates MAP kinase/ERK signalling and affects cell division and differentiation.

The number of other nonsynonymous somatic mutations was low in both APC and PCP and often consisted in cytosine to thymidine at CpG dinucleotides that resulted from spontaneous deamination rather than a pathogenetic mutation. In addition to the known mutation in *CTNNB1*, ACPs harboured isolated mutations in genes that are involved in transcriptional regulation, epigenetic regulation and DNA repair. Additional mutations in genes that are not listed in the Cancer Gene Census included genes involved in chromatin remodelling and regulation of transcription, cell cycle and DNA repair and cell adhesion. Many of these, however, were regarded as 'passenger' mutations that do not contribute to initiation or disease progression.

Unlike ACPs, PCPs did not show mutations in any other genes listed in the Cancer Gene Census but had isolated mutations in genes with potential roles in cancer including ones encoding chromatin remodelling factors and cell adhesion molecules and one (KIAA1549) that is fused to *BRAF* in most cases of pilocytic astrocytoma. Such mutations, like some of those found in ACPs, may also be 'passenger' mutations.

Targeted genotyping in a validation cohort of 98 CPs belonging to 95 different patients confirmed the results of the discovery cohort and showed BRAF V600E in 34 of the 36 PCPs. Sequencing results were further validated in 39 PCPs from 36 patients and 59 APCs using immunohistochemistry with an antibody VE1 that selectively recognises the mutant epitope BRAF V600E and an antibody directed against β-catenin. PCPs bearing the substitution BRAF V600E showed widespread immunoreactivity in squamous cells, whilst inflammatory and stromal cells were negative. The evidence of *BRAF* mutations in PCP opens new possibilities in the treatment of this tumour with BRAF inhibitors that are already in use for other forms of cancer such as melanoma (Ribas and Flaherty 2011) and hairy cell leukaemias (Dietrich et al. 2012). More recently, Larkin and colleagues (2014) observed the coexistence of BRAFV600E and *CTNNB1* in two of the 16 ACPs suggesting an overlap between PCPs and ACPs.

Acknowledgements Dr. Cynthia Andoniadou is acknowledged for her comments on this manuscript and for preparing Fig. 2.11.

References

Ackland FM, Stanhope R, Preece MA (1987) Cushing's disease and craniopharyngioma. Arch Dis Child 62:1077–1078

Adamson TE, Wiestler OD, Kleihues P, Yasargil MG (1990) Correlation of clinical and pathological features in surgically treated craniopharyngiomas. J Neurosurg 73:12–17

Agozzino L, Ferraraccio F, Accardo M et al (2006) Morphological and ultrastructural findings of prognostic impact in craniopharyngiomas. Ultrastruct Pathol 30(3):143–150

Akachi K et al (1987) Malignant changes in a craniopharyngioma. No Shinkei Geka 15(8):843–848

Alison MR, Murphy G, Leedham S (2008) Stem cells and cancer: a deadly mix. Cell Tissue Res 331(1):109–124

Alomari AK, Kelley BJ, Damisah E et al (2015) Craniopharyngioma arising in a Rathke's cleft cyst: case report. J Neurosurg Pediatr 15(3):250–254

Alvarez-Medina R, Le Dreau G, Ros M, Marti E (2009) Hedgehog activation is required upstream of Wnt signalling to control neural progenitor proliferation. Development 136(19):3301–3309

Andoniadou CL, Signore M, Sajedi E et al (2007) Lack of the murine homeobox gene Hesx1 leads to a posterior transformation of the anterior forebrain. Development 134(8):1499–1508

Andoniadou CL, Gaston-Massuet C, Reddy R, Schneider RP, Blasco MA, Le Tissier P, Jacques TS, Pevny LH, Dattani MT, Martinez-Barbera JP (2012) Identification of novel pathways involved in the pathogenesis of human adamantinomatous craniopharyngioma. Acta Neuropathol 124(2):259–271

Andoniadou CL, Matsushima D, Mousavy Gharavy SN et al (2013) Sox2(+) stem/progenitor cells in the adult mouse pituitary support organ homeostasis and have tumor-inducing potential. Cell Stem Cell 13(4):433–445

Aquilina K, O'Brien DF, Farrell MA et al (2006) Primary cerebellopontine angle craniopharyngioma in a patient with Gardner syndrome. Case report and review of the literature. J Neurosurg 105(2):330–333

Aquilina K, Merchant TE, Rodriguez-Galindo C et al (2010) Malignant transformation of irradiated craniopharyngioma in children: report of 2 cases. J Neurosurg Pediatr 5(2):155–161

Asa SL, Kovacs K, Bilbao JM et al (1981) Immunohistochemical localization of keratin in craniopharyngiomas and squamous cell nests of the human pituitary. Acta Neuropathol 54(3):257–260

Asari J, Yamanobe K, Sasaki T et al (1987) A case of prolactinoma associated with craniopharyngioma. No Shinkei Geka 15:1313–1318

Banczerowski P, Bálint K, Sipos L (2007) Temporal extradural ectopic craniopharyngioma. Case report. J Neurosurg 107(1):178–180

Barbounis V, Goutas N, Efremidis A (2013) Coexistence of intracranial germ cell tumor and craniopharyngioma in an adolescent: case report and review of the literature. Int J Clin Exp Med 6(3):211–218

Barker N, Ridgway RA, van Es JH et al (2009) Crypt stem cells as the cells-of-origin of intestinal cancer. Nature 457(7229):608–611

Barkhoudarian G, Laws ER (2013) Craniopharyngioma: history. Pituitary 16(1):1–8

Beaty NB, Ahn E (2014) Images in clinical medicine. Adamantinomatous craniopharyngioma containing teeth. N Engl J Med 370(9):860

Belza J (1966) Double midline intracranial tumors of vestigial origin: contiguous intrasellar chordoma and suprasellar craniopharyngioma. Case report. J Neurosurg 25:199–204

Bernstein ML, Buchino JJ. (1983) The histologic similarity between craniopharyngioma and odontogenic lesions: a reappraisal. Oral Surg Oral Med Oral Pathol. 56(5):502–11. PubMed PMID: 6196702

Bhattacharjee MB, Armstrong DD, Vogel H, Cooley LD (1997) Cytogenetic analysis of 120 primary pediatric brain tumors and literature review. Cancer Genet Cytogenet 97(1):39–53

Bijlsma MF, Roelink H (2010) Non-cell-autonomous signaling by Shh in tumors: challenges and opportunities for therapeutic targets. Expert Opin Ther Targets 14(7):693–702

Bikmaz K, Guerrero CA, Dammers R et al (2009) Ectopic recurrence of craniopharyngiomas: case report. Neurosurgery 64(2):E382–E383

Boongird A, Laothamatas J, Larbcharoensub N, Phudhichareonrat S (2009) Malignant craniopharyngioma: case report and review of the literature. Neuropathology 29(5):591–596

Bozbuga M, Turan Suslu H, Hicdonmez T, Bayindir C (2011) Primary cerebellopontine angle craniopharyngioma in a patient with Gardner syndrome. J Clin Neurosci 18(2):300–301

Brastianos PK, Taylor-Weiner A, Manley PE et al (2014) Exome sequencing identifies BRAF mutations in papillary craniopharyngiomas. Nat Genet 46(2):161–165

Broggi G, Franzini A, Cajola L, Pluchino F (1994) Cell kinetic investigations in craniopharyngioma: preliminary results and considerations. Pediatr Neurosurg 21(Suppl 1):21–23

Burghaus S, Holsken A, Buchfelder M et al (2010) A tumor-specific cellular environment at the brain invasion border of adamantinomatous craniopharyngiomas. Virchows Arch 456:287–300

Buslei R, Nolde M, Hofmann B et al (2005) Common mutations of beta-catenin in adamantinomatous craniopharyngiomas but not in other tumours originating from the sellar region. Acta Neuropathol 109(6):589–597

Buslei R, Holsken A, Hofmann B et al (2007) Nuclear beta-catenin accumulation associates with epithelial morphogenesis in craniopharyngiomas. Acta Neuropathol 113(5):585–590

Caceres A, Reitman AJ, Tomita T (2005) Craniopharyngioma and Cushing disease: case report. J Neurosurg 102:318–321

Campanini ML, Colli LM, Paixao BM et al (2010) CTNNB1 gene mutations, pituitary transcription factors, and MicroRNA expression involvement in the pathogenesis of adamantinomatous craniopharyngiomas. Horm Cancer 1(4):187–196

Cao J, Lin JP, Yang LX, Chen K, Huang ZS (2010) Expression of aberrant beta-catenin and impaired p63 in craniopharyngiomas. Br J Neurosurg 24(3):249–256

Caretti V, Sewing AC, Lagerweij T et al (2014) Human pontine glioma cells can induce murine tumors. Acta Neuropathol 127(6):897–909

Castinetti F, Davis SW, Brue T, Camper SA (2011) Pituitary stem cell update and potential implications for treating hypopituitarism. Endocr Rev 32(4):453–471

Chen H, Zhou L, Luo L et al (2013) Giant cranionasal and cystic-solid craniopharyngioma associated with extensive bone erosion and ossification. J Craniofac Surg 24(4):e398–e401

Clarke MF, Fuller M (2006) Stem cells and cancer: two faces of eve. Cell 124(6):1111–1115

Critchley M & Ironside RN (1926) The pituitary adenamantinomata 49(4):437–481

Crotty TB, Scheithauer BW, Young WF Jr et al (1995) Papillary craniopharyngioma: a clinicopathological study of 48 cases. J Neurosurg 83(2):206–214

Cushing H (1932) Intracranial tumors. Charles C Thomas, Baltimore

Cusimano MD, Kovacs K, Bilbao JM et al (1988) Suprasellar craniopharyngioma associated with hyperprolactinemia, pituitary lactotroph hyperplasia, and microprolactinoma. Case report. J Neurosurg 69:620–623

Davis SW, Mortensen AH, Camper SA (2011) Birthdating studies reshape models for pituitary gland cell specification. Dev Biol 352(2):215–227

de Almeida JP, Sherman JH, Salvatori R, Quinones-Hinojosa A (2010) Pituitary stem cells: review of the literature and current understanding. Neurosurgery 67(3):770–780

Demehri S, Turkoz A, Kopan R (2009) Epidermal Notch1 loss promotes skin tumorigenesis by impacting the stromal microenvironment. Cancer Cell 16(1):55–66

Deschene ER, Myung P, Rompolas P et al (2014) β-Catenin activation regulates tissue growth non-cell autonomously in the hair stem cell niche. Science 343(6177):1353–1356

Dietrich S, Glimm H, Andrulis M et al (2012) BRAF inhibition in refractory hairy-cell leukemia. N Engl J Med 366:2038–2040

Duò D, Gasverde S, Benech F et al (2003) MIB-1 immunoreactivity in craniopharyngiomas: a clinico-pathological analysis. Clin Neuropathol 22(5):229–234

Ebrahimi A, Honegger J, Schluesener H, Schittenhelm J (2013) Osteonectin expression in surrounding stroma of craniopharyngiomas: association with recurrence rate and brain infiltration. Int J Surg Pathol 21(6):591–598

Elmaci L, Kurtkaya-Yapicier O, Ekinci G et al (2002) Metastatic papillary craniopharyngioma: case study and study of tumor angiogenesis. Neuro Oncol 4(2):123–128

Erfurth EM, Holmer H, Fjalldal SB (2013) Mortality and morbidity in adult craniopharyngioma. Pituitary 16:46–55

Fauquier T, Rizzoti K, Dattani M et al (2008) SOX2-expressing progenitor cells generate all of the major cell types in the adult mouse pituitary gland. Proc Natl Acad Sci U S A 105(8):2907–2912

Finzi G, Cerati M, Marando A et al (2014) Mixed pituitary adenoma/craniopharyngioma: clinical, morphological, immunohistochemical and ultrastructural study of a case, review of the literature, and pathogenetic and nosological considerations. Pituitary 17(1):53–59

Florio T (2011) Adult pituitary stem cells: from pituitary plasticity to adenoma development. Neuroendocrinology 94(4):256–277

Frangou EM, Tynan JR, Robinson CA et al (2009) Metastatic craniopharyngioma: case report and literature review. Childs Nerv Syst 25(9):1143–1147

Frazier CH, Alpers BJ (1931) Adamantinoma of the craniopharyngeal duct. Arch Neurol Psychiatry 26:905–965

Gao S, Shi X, Wang Y, Qian H, Liu C (2011) Malignant transformation of craniopharyngioma: case report and review of the literature. J Neurooncol 103(3):719–725

Garcia-Lavandeira M, Quereda V, Flores I et al (2009) A GRFa2/Prop1/stem (GPS) cell niche in the pituitary. PLoS One 4(3):e4815

Garcia-Lavandeira M, Saez C, Diaz-Rodriguez E et al (2012) Craniopharyngiomas express embryonic stem cell markers (SOX2, OCT4, KLF4, and SOX9) as pituitary stem cells but do not coexpress RET/GFRA3 receptors. J Clin Endocrinol Metab 97(1):E80–E87

Gaston-Massuet C, Andoniadou CL, Signore M et al (2011) Increased Wingless (Wnt) signaling in pituitary progenitor/stem cells gives rise to pituitary tumors in mice and humans. Proc Natl Acad Sci U S A 108(28):11482–11487

Gautier A, Godbout A, Grosheny C et al (2012) Markers of recurrence and long-term morbidity in craniopharyngioma: a systematic analysis of 171 patients. J Clin Endocrinol Metab 97(4):1258–1267

Ghatak NR, Hirano A, Zimmerman HM (1971) Ultrastructure of a craniopharyngioma. Cancer 27:1465–1475

Giangaspero F, Burger PC, Osborne DR (1984) Suprasellar papillary squamous epithelioma ("papillary craniopharyngioma"). Am J Surg Pathol 8:57–64

Gibson P, Tong Y, Robinson G et al (2010) Subtypes of medulloblastoma have distinct developmental origins. Nature 468(7327):1095–1099

Gleiberman AS, Michurina T, Encinas JM et al (2008) Genetic approaches identify adult pituitary stem cells. Proc Natl Acad Sci U S A 105(17):6332–6337

Gökalp HZ, Mertol T (1990) Cerebellopontine angle craniopharyngioma. Neurochirurgia (Stuttg) 33(1):20–21

Gokden M, Mrak RE (2009) Pituitary adenoma with craniopharyngioma component. Hum Pathol 40(8):1189–1193

Goldberg GM, Eshbaugh DE (1960) Squamous cell nests of the pituitary gland as related to the origin of craniopharyngiomas: a study of their presence in the newborn and infants up kato age four. Arch Pathol 70:293–299

Gong J, Zhang H, Xing S et al (2014) High expression levels of CXCL12 and CXCR4 predict recurrence of adamantinomatous craniopharyngiomas in children. Cancer Biomark 14(4): 241–251

Gorski GK, McMorrow LE, Donaldson MH, Freed M (1992) Multiple chromosomal abnormalities in a case of craniopharyngioma. Cancer Genet Cytogenet 60:212–213

Griffin CA, Long PP, Carson BS, Brem H (1992) Chromosome abnormalities in low-grade central nervous system tumors. Cancer Genet Cytogenet 60(1):67–73

Guaraldi F, Prencipe N, di Giacomo V et al (2013) Association of craniopharyngioma and pituitary adenoma. Endocrine 44(1):59–65

Gupta K, Kuhn MJ, Shevlin DW, Wacaser LE (1999) Metastatic craniopharyngioma. AJNR Am J Neuroradiol 20(6):1059–1060

Gupta DK, Ojha BK, Sarkar C et al (2006) Recurrence in craniopharyngiomas: analysis of clinical and histological features. J Clin Neurosci 13(4):438–442

Han SJ, Rolston JD, Jahangiri A, Aghi MK (2014) Rathke's cleft cysts: review of natural history and surgical outcomes. J Neurooncol 117(2):197–203

Harris BT, Horoupian DS, Tse V, Herrick MK (1999) Melanotic craniopharyngioma: a report of two cases. Acta Neuropathol 98(4):433–436

Harrison MJ, Morgello S, Post KD (1994) Epithelial cystic lesions of the sellar and parasellar region: a continuum of ectodermal derivatives? J Neurosurg 80(6):1018–1025

He TC, Sparks AB, Rago C et al (1998) Identification of c-MYC as a target of the APC pathway. Science 281(5382):1509–1512

Herbst RS (2004) Review of epidermal growth factor receptor biology. Int J Radiat Oncol Biol Phys 59(2 Suppl):21–26

Herbst RS, Fukuoka M, Baselga J (2004) Gefitinib – a novel targeted approach to treating cancer. Nat Rev Cancer 4(12):956–965

Hofmann BM, Kreutzer J, Saeger W et al (2006) Nuclear beta-catenin accumulation as reliable marker for the differentiation between cystic craniopharyngiomas and rathke cleft cysts: a clinico-pathologic approach. Am J Surg Pathol 30(12):1595–1603

Holsken A, Kreutzer J, Hofmann BM et al (2009) Target gene activation of the Wnt signaling pathway in nuclear beta-catenin accumulating cells of adamantinomatous craniopharyngiomas. Brain Pathol 19(3):357–364

Holsken A, Gebhardt M, Buchfelder M et al (2011) EGFR signaling regulates tumor cell migration in craniopharyngiomas. Clin Cancer Res 17(13):4367–4377

Holsken A, Stache C, Schlaffer SM et al (2014) Adamantinomatous craniopharyngiomas express tumor stem cell markers in cells with activated Wnt signaling: further evidence for the existence of a tumor stem cell niche? Pituitary 17(6):546–556

Honegger J, Renner C, Fahlbusch R, Adams EF (1997) Progesterone receptor gene expression in craniopharyngiomas and evidence for biological activity. Neurosurgery 41:1359–1364

Hunter IJ (1955) Squamous metaplasia of cells of the anterior pituitary gland. J Pathol Bacteriol 69:141–145

Hussain I, Eloy JA, Carmel PW, Liu JK (2013) Molecular oncogenesis of craniopharyngioma: current and future strategies for the development of targeted therapies. J Neurosurg 119(1):106–112

Inenaga C, Kakita A, Iwasaki Y, Yamatani K, Takahashi H (2004) Autopsy findings of a craniopharyngioma with a natural course over 60 years. Surg Neurol 61(6):536–540

Ingham PW, Placzek M (2006) Orchestrating ontogenesis: variations on a theme by sonic hedgehog. Nat Rev Genet 7(11):841–850

Ito M, Jamshidi J, Yamanaka K (2001) Does craniopharyngioma metastasize? Case report and review of the literature. Neurosurgery 48(4):933–935

Izumoto S, Suzuki T, Kinoshita M et al (2005) Immunohistochemical detection of female sex hormone receptors in craniopharyngiomas: correlation with clinical and histologic features. Surg Neurol 63(520–525):2005

Jayakody SA, Andoniadou CL, Gaston-Massuet C et al (2012) SOX2 regulates the hypothalamic-pituitary axis at multiple levels. J Clin Invest 122(10):3635–3646

Jho EH, Zhang T, Domon C et al (2002) Wnt/beta-catenin/Tcf signaling induces the transcription of Axin2, a negative regulator of the signaling pathway. Mol Cell Biol 22(4):1172–1183

Jiang RS, Wu CY, Jan YJ, Hsu CY (1998) Primary ethmoid sinus craniopharyngioma: a case report. J Laryngol Otol 112(4):403–405

Jin G, Hao S, Xie J, Mi R, Liu F (2013) Collision tumors of the sella: coexistence of pituitary adenoma and craniopharyngioma in the sellar region. World J Surg Oncol 7(11):178

Jones RT, Abedalthagafi MS, Brahmandam M et al (2015) Cross-reactivity of the BRAF VE1 antibody with epitopes in axonemal dyneins leads to staining of cilia. Mod Pathol 28(4): 596–606

Karavitaki N, Brufani C, Warner JT et al (2005) Craniopharyngiomas in children and adults: systematic analysis of 121 cases with long-term follow-up. Clin Endocrinol (Oxf) 62:397–409

Karavitaki N, Scheithauer BW, Watt J et al (2008) Collision lesions of the sella: coexistence of craniopharyngioma with gonadotroph adenoma and of Rathke's cleft cyst with corticotroph adenoma. Pituitary 11:317–323

Karnes PS, Tran TN, Cui MY et al (1992) Cytogenetic analysis of 39 pediatric central nervous system tumors. Cancer Genet Cytogenet 59:12–19

Kasai H, Hirano A, Llena JF, Kawamoto K (1997) A histopathological study of craniopharyngioma with special reference to its stroma and surrounding tissue. Brain Tumor Pathol 14(1):41–45

Kato K, Nakatani Y, Kanno H et al (2004) Possible linkage between specific histological structures and aberrant reactivation of the Wnt pathway in adamantinomatous craniopharyngioma. J Pathol 203(3):814–821

Kawamata T, Kubo O, Kamikawa S, Hori T (2002) Ectopic clival craniopharyngioma. Acta Neurochir (Wien) 144(11):1221–1224

Kawamata T, Kubo O, Hori T (2005) Histological findings at the boundary of craniopharyngiomas. Brain Tumor Pathol 22(2):75–78

Kayaselçuk F, Zorludemir S, Gümürdühü D et al (2002) PCNA and Ki-67 in central nervous system tumors: correlation with the histological type and grade. J Neurooncol 57(2):115–121

Kelberman D, de Castro SC, Huang S et al (2008) SOX2 plays a critical role in the pituitary, forebrain, and eye during human embryonic development. J Clin Endocrinol Metab 93(5):1865–1873

Kepes JJ (1978) Transitional cell tumor of the pituitary gland developing from a Rathke's cleft cyst. Cancer 41;337–343

Kikuchi K, Ito S, Inoue H, González-Alva P et al (2012) Immunohistochemical expression of podoplanin in so-called hard α-keratin-expressing tumors, including calcifying cystic odontogenic tumor, craniopharyngioma, and pilomatrixoma. J Oral Sci 54(2):165–175

Kim SK, Wang KC, Shin SH et al (2001) Radical excision of pediatric craniopharyngioma: recurrence pattern and prognostic factors. Childs Nerv Syst 17(9):531–536; discussion 537

Kim JS, Crooks H, Dracheva T et al (2002) Oncogenic beta-catenin is required for bone morphogenetic protein 4 expression in human cancer cells. Cancer Res 62(10):2744–2748

Kim MS, Kim YS, Lee HK et al (2014) Primary intracranial ectopic craniopharyngioma in a patient with probable Gardner's syndrome. J Neurosurg 120(2):337–341

Kim JH, Paulus W, Heim S (2015) BRAF V600E mutation is a useful marker for differentiating Rathke's cleft cyst with squamous metaplasia from papillary craniopharyngioma. J Neurooncol 123(1):189–191

Kode A, Manavalan JS, Mosialou I et al (2014) Leukaemogenesis induced by an activating beta-catenin mutation in osteoblasts. Nature 506(7487):240–244

Kristopaitis T, Thomas C, Petruzzelli GJ, Lee JM (2000) Malignant craniopharyngioma. Arch Pathol Lab Med 124(9):1356–1360

Kurosaki M, Saeger W, Lüdecke DK (2001) Immunohistochemical localisation of cytokeratins in craniopharyngioma. Acta Neurochir (Wien) 143(2):147

Kusama K, Katayama Y, Oba K et al (2005) Expression of hard alpha-keratins in pilomatrixoma, craniopharyngioma, and calcifying odontogenic cyst. Am J Clin Pathol 123(3):376–381

Larkin SJ, Ansorge O (2013) Pathology and pathogenesis of craniopharyngiomas. Pituitary 16(1):9–17

Larkin SJ, Preda V, Karavitaki N et al (2014) BRAF V600E mutations are characteristic for papillary craniopharyngioma and may coexist with CTNNB1-mutated adamantinomatous craniopharyngioma. Acta Neuropathol 127(6):927–929. doi: 10.1007/s00401-014-1270-6. Epub 2014 Apr 9. PubMed PMID: 24715106; PubMed Central PMCID: PMC4024131

Laurent-Puig P, Lievre A, Blons H (2009) Mutations and response to epidermal growth factor receptor inhibitors. Clin Cancer Res 15(4):1133–1139

Lauriola L, Doglietto F, Novello M et al (2011) De novo malignant craniopharyngioma: case report and literature review. J Neurooncol 103(2):381–386

Le BH, Towfighi J, Kapadia SB, Lopes MB (2007) Comparative immunohistochemical assessment of craniopharyngioma and related lesions. Endocr Pathol 18(1):23–30

Lee DK, Jung HW, Kim DG et al (2001) Postoperative spinal seeding of craniopharyngioma. Case report. J Neurosurg 94(4):617–620

Lee YH, Kim SD, Lim DJ et al (2009) Isolated petroclival craniopharyngioma with aggressive skull base destruction. Yonsei Med J 50(5):729–731

Lefranc F, Chevalier C, Vinchon M et al (2003) Characterization of the levels of expression of retinoic acid receptors, galectin-3, macrophage migration inhibitory factor and p53 in 51 adamantinomatous craniopharyngiomas. J Neurosurg 98:145–153

Lefranc F, Mijatovic T, Decaestecker C et al (2005) Monitoring the expression profiles of integrins and adhesion/growth-regulatory galectins in adamantinomatous craniopharyngiomas: their ability to regulate tumor adhesiveness to surrounding tissue and their contribution to prognosis. Neurosurgery 56(4):763–776

Lepore DA, Roeszler K, Wagner J et al (2005) Identification and enrichment of colony-forming cells from the adult murine pituitary. Exp Cell Res 308(1):166–176

Lindholm J, Nielsen EH (2009) Craniopharyngioma: historical notes. Pituitary 12(4):352–359

Losa M, Vimercati A, Acerno S et al (2004) Correlation between clinical characteristics and proliferative activity in patients with craniopharyngioma. J Neurol Neurosurg Psychiatry 75(6):889–892

Lubansu A, Ruchoux MM, Brotchi J et al (2003) Cathepsin B, D and K expression in adamantinomatous craniopharyngiomas relates to their levels of differentiation as determined by the patterns of retinoic acid receptor expression. Histopathology 43:563–572

Lujambio A, Akkari L, Simon J et al (2013) Non-cell-autonomous tumor suppression by p53. Cell 153(2):449–460

Malik JM, Cosgrove GR, VandenBerg SR (1992) Remote recurrence of craniopharyngioma in the epidural space. Case report. J Neurosurg 77(5):804–807

Matsushima T, Fukui M, Ohta M et al (1980) Ciliated and goblet cells in craniopharyngioma. Acta Neuropathol 50:199–205

Mendelsohn J, Baselga J (2000) The EGF receptor family as targets for cancer therapy. Oncogene 19(56):6550–6565

Moshkin O, Scheithauer BW, Syro LV et al (2009) Collision tumors of the sella: craniopharyngioma and silent pituitary adenoma subtype 3: case report. Endocr Pathol 20(1):50–55

Mott FW, Barrett JOW (1899) Three cases of tumor of the third ventricle. Arch Neurol (Lond) 1:417–440

Mukherjee JJ, Islam N, Kaltsas G et al (1997) Clinical, radiological and pathological features of patients with Rathke's cleft cysts: tumors that may recur. J Clin Endocrinol Metab 82:2357–2362

Müller HL (2014) Craniopharyngioma. Endocr Rev 35(3):513–543

Müller HL, Gebhardt U, Schröder S et al (2010) Analyses of treatment variables for patients with childhood craniopharyngioma–results of the multicenter prospective trial KRANIOPHARYNGEOM 2000 after three years of follow-up. Horm Res Paediatr 73:175–180

Musani V, Gorry P, Basta-Juzbasic A et al (2006) Mutation in exon 7 of PTCH deregulates SHH/PTCH/SMO signaling: possible linkage to WNT. Int J Mol Med 17(5):755–759

Nelson GA, Bastian FO, Schlitt M, White RL (1988) Malignant transformation in craniopharyngioma. Neurosurgery 22(2):427–429

Netsky MG (1988) Epidermoid tumors. Review of the literature. Surg Neurol 29(6):477–483

Nguyen LV, Vanner R, Dirks P, Eaves CJ (2012) Cancer stem cells: an evolving concept. Nat Rev Cancer 12(2):133–143

Nicolas M, Wolfer A, Raj K et al (2003) Notch1 functions as a tumor suppressor in mouse skin. Nat Genet 33(3):416–421

Nishi T, Kuratsu J, Takeshima H et al (1999) Prognostic significance of the MIB-1 labeling index for patients with craniopharyngiomas. Int J Mol Med 3:157–161

Nishio S, Mizuno J, Barrow DL et al (1987) Pituitary tumors composed of adenohypophysial adenoma and Rathke's cleft cyst elements: a clinicopathological study. Neurosurgery 21(3):371–377

Novegno F, Di Rocco F, Colosimo C Jr et al (2002) Ectopic recurrences of craniopharyngioma. Childs Nerv Syst 18(9–10):468–473

Oikonomou E, Barreto DC, Soares B et al (2005) Beta-catenin mutations in craniopharyngiomas and pituitary adenomas. J Neurooncol 73(3):205–209

Oka H, Kawano N, Yagishita S et al (1997) Ciliated craniopharyngioma indicates histogenetic relationship to Rathke cleft epithelium. Clin Neuropathol 16(2):103–106. PubMed PMID: 9101113

Okada T, Fujitsu K, Miyahara K et al (2010) Ciliated craniopharyngioma – case report and pathological study. Acta Neurochir (Wien) 152(2):303–306 discussion 307. doi:10.1007/s00701-009-0448-5. Epub 2009 Jul 21. PubMed PMID: 19626269

Ono M, Kuwano M (2006) Molecular mechanisms of epidermal growth factor receptor (EGFR) activation and response to gefitinib and other EGFR-targeting drugs. Clin Cancer Res 12(24):7242–7251

Ortega-Porcayo LA, Ponce-Gómez JA, Martínez-Moreno M et al (2015) Primary ectopic fronto-temporal craniopharyngioma. Int J Surg Case Rep 9:57–60

Pascual JM, Rosdolsky M, Prieto R et al (2015) Jakob Erdheim (1874–1937): father of hypophyseal-duct tumors (craniopharyngiomas). Virchows Arch 467(4):459–469

Paulus W, Stöckel C, Krauss J et al (1997) Odontogenic classification of craniopharyngiomas: a clinicopathological study of 54 cases. Histopathology 30(2):172–176

Paulus W, Honegger J, Keyvani K, Fahlbusch R (1999) Xanthogranuloma of the sellar region: a clinicopathological entity different from adamantinomatous craniopharyngioma. Acta Neuropathol 97(4):377–382

Petito CK, DeGirolami U, Earle KM (1976) Craniopharyngiomas: a clinical and pathological review. Cancer 37:1944–1952

Powers CJ, New KC, McLendon RE, Friedman AH, Fuchs HE (2007) Cerebellopontine angle craniopharyngioma: case report and literature review. Pediatr Neurosurg 43(2):158–163

Prabhakar V, Rao BD, Subramanyam MV (1971) Pituitary adenoma associated with craniopharyngioma. J Pathol 103:185–187

Prieto R, Pascual JM, Subhi-Issa I et al (2013) Predictive factors for craniopharyngioma recurrence: a systematic review and illustrative case report of a rapid recurrence. World Neurosurg 79(5–6):733–749

Proescholdt M, Merrill M, Stoerr EM et al (2011) Expression of carbonic anhydrase IX in craniopharyngiomas. J Neurosurg 115(4):796–801

Qi ST, Zhou J, Pan J et al (2012) Epithelial-mesenchymal transition and clinicopathological correlation in craniopharyngioma. Histopathology 61(4):711–725

Raghavan R, Dickey WT Jr et al (2000) Proliferative activity in craniopharyngiomas: clinicopathological correlations in adults and children. Surg Neurol 54(3):241–247; discussion 248
Ren X, Lin S, Wang Z et al (2012) Clinical, radiological, and pathological features of 24 atypical
intracranial epidermoid cysts. J Neurosurg 116(3):611–621
Ribas A, Flaherty KT (2011) BRAF targeted therapy changes the treatment paradigm in melanoma. Nat Rev Clin Oncol 8:426–433
Rickert CH, Paulus W (2003) Lack of chromosomal imbalances in adamantinomatous and papillary craniopharyngiomas. J Neurol Neurosurg Psychiatry 74(2):260–261
Rienstein S, Adams EF, Pilzer D et al (2003) Comparative genomic hybridization analysis of craniopharyngiomas. J Neurosurg 98:162–164
Rizzoti K, Akiyama H, Lovell-Badge R (2013) Mobilized adult pituitary stem cells contribute to
endocrine regeneration in response to physiological demand. Cell Stem Cell 13(4):419–432
Rodriguez FJ, Scheithauer BW, Tsunoda S et al (2007) The spectrum of malignancy in craniopharyngioma. Am J Surg Pathol 31(7):1020–1028
Romer JT, Kimura H, Magdaleno S et al (2004) Suppression of the Shh pathway using a small
molecule inhibitor eliminates medulloblastoma in Ptc1(+/−)p53(−/−) mice. Cancer Cell
6(3):229–240
Rubin LL, de Sauvage FJ (2006) Targeting the Hedgehog pathway in cancer. Nat Rev Drug Discov
5(12):1026–1033
Rudin CM, Hann CL, Laterra J et al (2009) Treatment of medulloblastoma with hedgehog pathway
inhibitor GDC-0449. N Engl J Med 361(12):1173–1178
Rushing EJ, Giangaspero F, Paulus W, Burger PC (2007) Craniopharyngioma. In: Louis DN,
Ohgaki H, Wiestler OD, Webster KC (eds) WHO classification of tumours of the central ner-
vous system, 3rd edn. World Health Organization Press, Geneva, pp 238–240
Salyer D, Carter D (1973) Squamous carcinoma arising in the pituitary gland. Cancer 31(3):713–718
Sargis RM, Wollmann RL, Pytel P (2009) A 59 year-old man with sellar lesion. Brain Pathol
19(1):161–162
Sarubi JC, Bei H, Adams EF et al (2001) Clonal composition of human adamantinomatous craniopharyngiomas and somatic mutation analyses of the patched (PTCH), Gsalpha and Gi2alpha
genes. Neurosci Lett 310:5–8
Schittenhelm J, Psaras T, Meyermann R et al (2010) Pituitary adenomas and craniopharyngiomas
are CDX2 negative neoplasms. Folia Neuropathol 48:75–80
Schweizer L, Capper D, Hölsken A et al (2015) BRAF V600E analysis for the differentiation
of papillary craniopharyngiomas and Rathke's cleft cysts. Neuropathol Appl Neurobiol
41(6):733–742. doi: 10.1111/nan.12201. Epub 2015 May 2. PubMed PMID: 25442675.
Seemayer TA, Blundell JS, Wiglesworth FW (1972) Pituitary craniopharyngioma with tooth formation. Cancer 29:423–430
Sekine S, Shibata T, Kokubu A et al (2002) Craniopharyngiomas of adamantinomatous type har-
bor beta-catenin gene mutations. Am J Pathol 161(6):1997–2001
Sekine S, Takata T, Shibata T et al (2004) Expression of enamel proteins and LEF1 in adamantinomatous craniopharyngioma: evidence for its odontogenic epithelial differentiation.
Histopathology 45(6):573–579
Shah GB, Bhaduri AS, Misra BK (2007) Ectopic craniopharyngioma of the fourth ventricle: case
report. Surg Neurol 68(1):96–98
Shapiro K, Till K, Grant DN. (1979) Craniopharyngiomas in childhood. A rational approach to
treatment. J Neurosurg. 50(5):617–23. PubMed PMID: 430156
Shin JL, Asa SL, Woodhouse LJ et al (1999) Cystic lesions of the pituitary: clinicopathologi-
cal features distinguishing craniopharyngioma, Rathke's cleft cyst, and arachnoid cyst. J Clin
Endocrinol Metab 84(11):3972–3982. PubMed PMID: 10566636
Shin K, Lee J, Guo N et al (2011) Hedgehog/Wnt feedback supports regenerative proliferation of
epithelial stem cells in bladder. Nature 472(7341):110–114
Sofela AA, Hettige S, Curran O, Bassi S (2014) Malignant transformation in craniopharyngiomas.
Neurosurgery 75(3):306–314

Solarski A, Panke ES, Panke TW (1978) Craniopharyngioma in the pineal gland. Arch Pathol Lab Med 102(9):490–491

Stache C, Hölsken A, Fahlbusch R et al (2014) Tight junction protein claudin-1 is differentially expressed in craniopharyngioma subtypes and indicates invasive tumor growth. Neuro Oncol 16(2):256–264

Stache C, Hölsken A, Schlaffer SM et al (2015) Insights into the infiltrative behavior of adamantinomatous craniopharyngioma in a new xenotransplant mouse model. Brain Pathol 25(1):1–10. doi: 10.1111/bpa.12148. Epub 2014 May 19. PubMed PMID:24716541

Sumida M, Uozumi T, Mukada K et al (1994) Rathke cleft cysts: correlation of enhanced MR and surgical findings. AJNR Am J Neuroradiol 15(3):525–532

Sun HI, Akgun E, Bicer A et al (2010) Expression of angiogenic factors in craniopharyngiomas: implications for tumor recurrence. Neurosurgery 66(4):744–750; discussion 750

Szeifert GT, Julow J, Slowik F et al (1990) Pathological changes in cystic craniopharyngiomas following intracavital 90yttrium treatment. Acta Neurochir (Wien) 102(1–2):14–18. PubMed PMID: 1689531

Tateyama H, Tada T, Okabe M et al (2001) Different keratin profiles in craniopharyngioma subtypes and ameloblastomas. Pathol Res Pract 197(11):735–742

Tena-Suck ML, Salinas-Lara C, Arce-Arellano RI et al (2006) Clinico-pathological and immunohistochemical characteristics associated to recurrence/regrowth of craniopharyngiomas. Clin Neurol Neurosurg 108(7):661–669

Tetsu O, McCormick F (1999) Beta-catenin regulates expression of cyclin D1 in colon carcinoma cells. Nature 398(6726):422–426

Thapar K, Stefaneanu L, Kovacs K et al (1994) Estrogen receptor gene expression in craniopharyngiomas: an in situ hybridization study. Neurosurgery 35:1012–1017

Theunissen JW, de Sauvage FJ (2009) Paracrine Hedgehog signaling in cancer. Cancer Res 69(15):6007–6010

Vankelecom H (2012) Pituitary stem cells drop their mask. Curr Stem Cell Res Ther 7(1):36–71

Vaquero J, Zurita M, de Oya S et al (1999) Expression of vascular permeability factor in craniopharyngioma. J Neurosurg 91(5):831–834

Vidal S, Kovacs K, Lloyd RV et al (2002) Angiogenesis in patients with craniopharyngiomas: correlation with treatment and outcome. Cancer 94:738–745

Virik K, Turner J, Garrick R, Sheehy JP (1999) Malignant transformation of craniopharyngioma. J Clin Neurosci 6(6):527–530

Visvader JE, Lindeman GJ (2012) Cancer stem cells: current status and evolving complexities. Cell Stem Cell 10(6):717–728

Wang W, Chen XD, Bai HM et al (2015) Malignant transformation of craniopharyngioma with detailed follow-up. Neuropathology 35(1):50–55

Weiner HL, Wisoff JH, Rosenberg ME et al (1994) Craniopharyngiomas: a clinicopathological analysis of factors predictive of recurrence and functional outcome. Neurosurgery 35(6):1001–1010

Wheatley T, Clark JD, Stewart S (1986) Craniopharyngioma with hyperprolactinaemia due to a prolactinoma. J Neurol Neurosurg Psychiatry 49:1305–1307

Xia Z, Liu W, Li S et al (2011) Expression of matrix metalloproteinase-9, type IV collagen and vascular endothelial growth factor in adamantinous craniopharyngioma. Neurochem Res 36(12):2346–2351

Xin W, Rubin MA, McKeever PE (2002) Differential expression of cytokeratins 8 and 20 distinguishes craniopharyngioma from rathke cleft cyst. Arch Pathol Lab Med 126(10):1174–1178

Xu J, You C, Zhang S et al (2006) Angiogenesis and cell proliferation in human craniopharyngioma xenografts in nude mice. J Neurosurg 105(Suppl 4):306–310

Xu J, Zhang S, You C et al (2007) Expression of human MCM6 and DNA Topo II alpha in craniopharyngiomas and its correlation with recurrence of the tumor. J Neurooncol 83(2):183–189. Epub 2007 Apr 5. PubMed PMID: 17410335

Yan Y, Tang WY, Yang G, Zhong D (2009) Isolated cerebellopontine angle craniopharyngioma. J Clin Neurosci 16(12):1655–1657

Yauch RL, Gould SE, Scales SJ et al (2008) A paracrine requirement for hedgehog signalling in cancer. Nature 455(7211):406–410

Yoshida A, Sen C, Asa SL, Rosenblum MK (2008) Composite pituitary adenoma and cranio-pharyngioma?: an unusual sellar neoplasm with divergent differentiation. Am J Surg Pathol 32(11):1736–1741

Yoshimoto M, de Toledo SR, da Silva NS et al (2004) Comparative genomic hybridization analysis of pediatric adamantinomatous craniopharyngiomas and a review of the literature. J Neurosurg 101(1 Suppl):85–90

Zada G, Lin N, Ojerholm E et al (2010) Craniopharyngioma and other cystic epithelial lesions of the sellar region: a review of clinical, imaging, and histopathological relationships. Neurosurg Focus 28(4):E4

Zhu L, Gibson P, Currle DS et al (2009) Prominin 1 marks intestinal stem cells that are susceptible to neoplastic transformation. Nature 457(7229):603–607

Zuhur SS, Müslüman AM, Tanık C et al (2011) MGMT immunoexpression in adamantinomatous craniopharyngiomas. Pituitary 14(4):323–327

Gennaro D'Anna, Marco Grimaldi, and Giuseppe Scotti

Abstract

The imaging finding in craniopharyngioma is related to the morphology and the structure of its two subtypes: Adamantinomatous craniopharyngioma is a cystic, partially calcific suprasellar mass, displacing the surrounding anatomical structures; after gadolinium administration, it demonstrates enhancement of the cystic wall. The papillary subtype is a mixed solid/cystic lesion, without calcifications, that inhomogeneously enhances after gadolinium administration. Important is differential diagnosis with other suprasellar lesions, as macroadenoma, astrocytoma, Rathke cleft cyst, or giant aneurysm.

3.1 Introduction

Two distinct imaging features characterize craniopharyngiomas, reflecting the morphology and the structure of the two most common subtypes: adamantinomatous and papillary (Lucas and Zada 2012). The adamantinomatous subtype is characterized by cyst formation and calcifications and is more common in children (Müller 2013). Conversely, the papillary one is more frequent in adults and is formed by papillary squamous epithelium. Calcifications or cystic components are generally less frequently present or are not detectable (Osborn 2012). Although the majority of craniopharyngiomas involve the suprasellar space, about half of the cases exhibit

G. D'Anna (✉)
Radiology Unit, Humanitas Mater Domini, Castellanza, VA, Italy
e-mail: gennaro.danna@gmail.com

M. Grimaldi • G. Scotti
Neuroradiology Unit, Humanitas Research Hospital, Rozzano, MI, Italy
e-mail: marco.grimaldi@humanitas.it; Giuseppe.scotti@humanitas.it

© Springer International Publishing Switzerland 2016
A. Lania et al. (eds.), *Diagnosis and Management of Craniopharyngiomas:
Key Current Topics*, DOI 10.1007/978-3-319-22297-4_3

55

intrasellar involvement (Karavitaki et al. 2006). Craniopharyngiomas may extend into the anterior, middle, or posterior fossa and may invade the floor or walls of the third ventricle (Van Effenterre and Boch 2002) (Fig. 3.1).

3.2   Imaging Technique

The sellar pathology is studied actually with computed tomography (CT) and magnetic resonance imaging (MRI). CT images are obtained, on the modern multislice scanner, with a volumetric scan with and without iodinated contrast material administration.

MRI scan is nowadays the "gold standard" in the imaging of the region: besides showing the lesion, it clearly shows the relationships between the tumor and the anatomical structures inside and outside the sellar region. An MRI scan of the sellar-parasellar region needs a high-field machine (1 T minimum) and includes both non-contrast and contrast-enhanced sequences. Slices are minimum 3 mm thick or less, exploring the region mainly with sagittal and coronal orientation. A standard protocol includes both T1W and T2W sequences on sagittal and coronal plane (optional is a fat saturated T1 sequence) followed by sagittal and coronal T1W images after intravenous gadolinium-based contrast administration. Other sequences (as diffusion, gradient echo) can be used in selected cases, when the diagnosis is not straightforward, or to try to identify calcifications.

3.3   General Features

Craniopharyngiomas generally appear as a solitary suprasellar mass lesion, of variable size, up to 5 cm in diameter (Curran and O'Connor 2005). As it grows, the mass may invade the anterior, middle, and posterior fossae. Tumor growth usually displaces the anterior portion of the circle of Willis, as seen on MR angiography. The pituitary gland is unaffected and the sellar volume is normal. Purely intrasellar infradiaphragmatic craniopharyngiomas are rarer, and the pituitary gland, compressed and dislocated, is usually clearly separated from the neoplastic mass. The sella turcica may be enlarged by the presence of the tumor in these cases. The brain tissue adjacent to the lesion may be normal, or it may show signal abnormalities on T2W and FLAIRW images, related to edema. Hydrocephalus may be present, due to third ventricle compression from below. The most important goal of the imaging of craniopharyngiomas is the identification of the relationships between tumor and adjacent structures. One of the most frequent symptoms is visual loss, that is, related to compression of the optic system by the upwards growing lesion: compression and/or stretching of a single or multiple segments (Prieto et al. 2015) may take place. Other important features detectable on MRI are the displacement and eventual encasement of the branches of the polygon of Willis. CT or MR angiography may be useful to detect the displacement and to depict the relationship of the craniopharyngioma with the arterial branches. MRI is also very useful to preoperatively detect the position of the pituitary stalk and to measure the length of the optic nerves and by consequence the position of the chiasm. This data may be useful to the surgeon in choosing the best surgical approach in any given case.

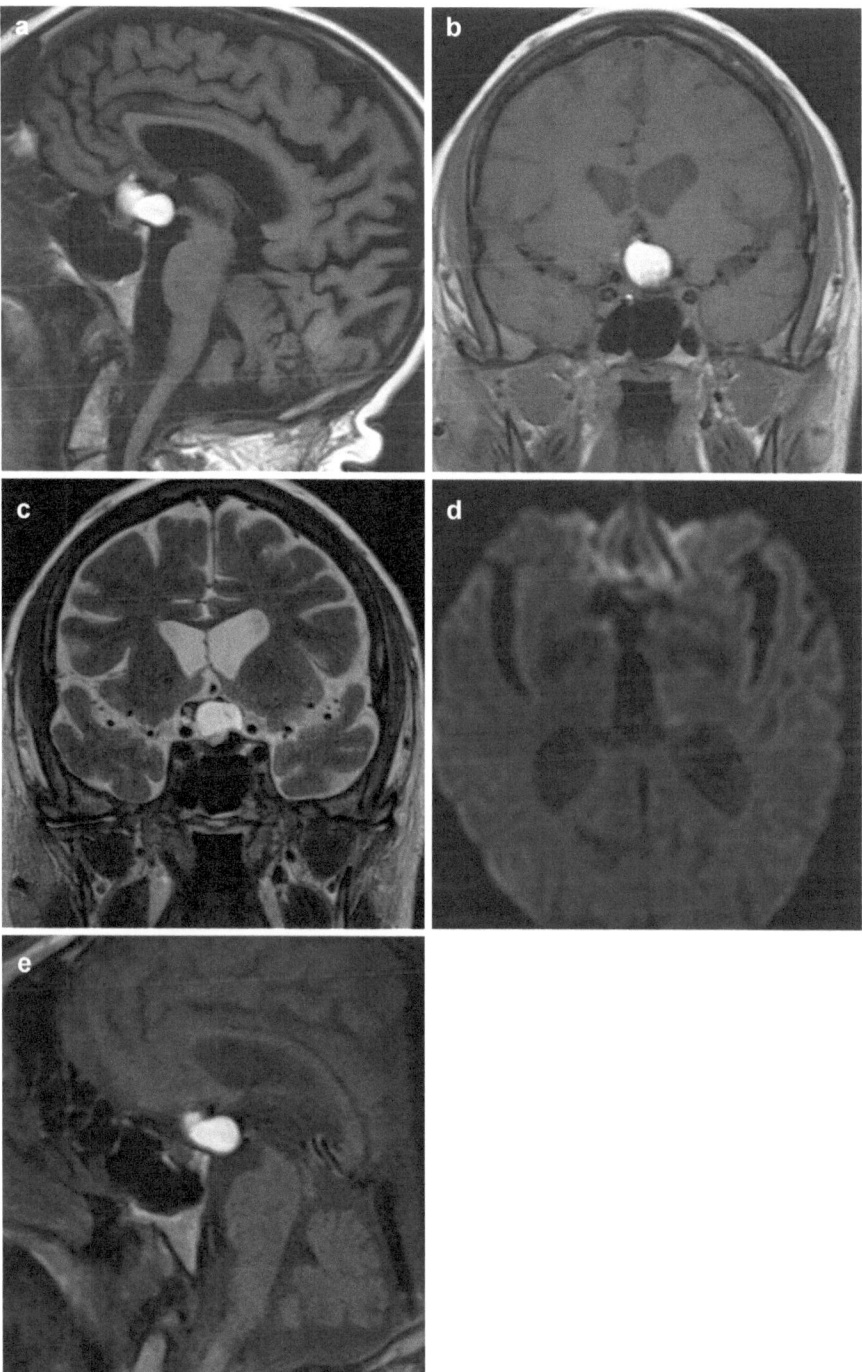

Fig. 3.1   Adamantinomatous craniopharyngioma. (**a**, **b**) Sagittal and coronal T1WI demonstrates hyperintense suprasellar lesion, with third ventricle compression; in (**c**), coronal T2WI shows hyperintense signal of the lesion, without restricted diffusion on DWI (**d**). After administration of contrast media, on sagittal T1WI (**e**), no enhancement was noted

3.4   Adamantinous Subtype

The tumor shows usually a cystic component, calcifications are common, and the cystic wall enhances after contrast administration. Adamantinomatous craniopharyngiomas arise from anywhere along the primitive craniopharyngeal duct, but 90–95 % have a suprasellar component; pure intrasellar tumors are rare, seen in 5 % or fewer of cases (Fig. 3.1).

On CT, a hypodense suprasellar cystic mass is depicted. A variable amount of intratumoral and/or cyst wall calcifications is usually present (up to 60 %of cases) (Sartoretti-Schefer et al. 1997; Borges 2009; Karavitaki et al. 2006; Weiner et al. 1994) (Fig. 3.2).

On MRI a uni- or multilocular cystic mass, with a small solid nodulation is showed. When present the solid tumor portion is iso/hypointense on precontrast T1-weighted images and exhibits heterogeneous hyper-/hypointensity on T2W/FLAIRW images (Ahmadi et al. 1992). The single or multiloculated cystic portion shows predominantly high intensity on T1-weighted image: this characteristic finding is related to the presence of cholesterol, keratin, and desquamated squamous epithelium in the cystic fluid, described as "machine oil" sign (Ginat and Meyers 2012; Zada et al. 2010). The inhomogeneous T2 signal is also related to the presence of wet keratine nodules. The thin wall of the cyst shows enhancement on T1-weighted images after contrast administration, while the solid portion shows inhomogeneous enhancement due to necrotic components (Choi et al. 2007). As suggested by A. Osborn, adamantinomatous craniopharyngiomas follow a "rule of ninety": 90 % are mixed cystic/solid, 90 % are calcified, and 90 % enhanced (Osborn 2012).

On MR spectroscopy, the lesion may show a broad lipid spectrum, due to the large presence of cholesterol.

On DWI, no restricted diffusion signal is shown in the cystic portion.

Although MR isn't sensitive to demonstrate calcifications, they may be depicted on gradient echo (GRE) images, as susceptibility artifacts within the tumor tissue.

3.5   Papillary Subtype

The papillary subtype is more frequent in adults. The lesion typically appears as a suprasellar solid or solid/cystic mass. Cysts are rarely present and small in size (Crotty et al. 1995); calcifications are absent. On CT imaging, an isodense suprasellar lesion is seen, spheric-ovoidal in shape, without calcifications (Tsuda et al. 1997). On MRI, the lesion shows an iso- to slightly hypointense T1 signal. On T2WI the signal is markedly hyperintense; foci of less intensity may be present (Sartoretti-Schefer et al. 1997; Zada et al. 2010). The rare cystic components show hypointense signal in T1WI and high signal in T2WI. After contrast administration, the solid portion inhomogeneously enhances as the cyst walls. On MR spectroscopy, the lipid spectrum is absent (Fig. 3.3).

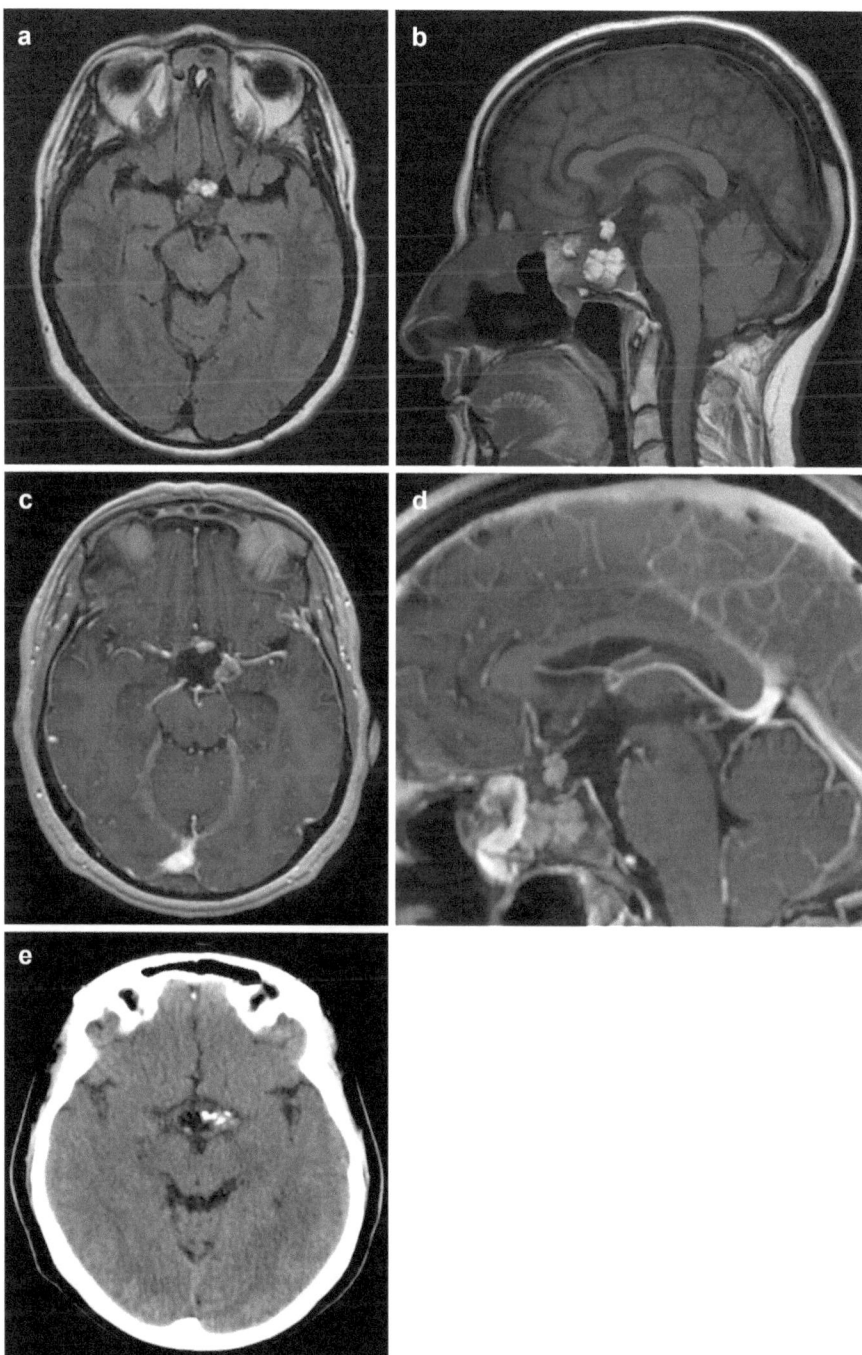

Fig. 3.2 Recurrent adamantinomatous craniopharyngioma. (**a**) Transverse FLAIR shows supra-sellar lesion with disomogeneous hyperintense portions. In (**b**) the lesion shows invasion of sphenoidal sinus, with many portions hyperintense. No enhancement after gadolinium administration (**c**, **d**). CT scan demonstrates many calcification on the left side of the lesion (**e**)

3.6　Differential Diagnosis

Differential diagnosis of craniopharyngioma, due to its intrinsic characteristics and location, must take into consideration the following lesions:

- *Rathke cleft cyst* (RCC): RCCs usually don't exhibit calcifications and are more homogeneous, without solid nodules and wall enhancement after contrast media administration. Nevertheless, small RCCs may be indistinguishable from craniopharyngiomas (Choi et al. 2007; Osborn and Preece 2006). Kunii et al. founded that both the ADC and relative ADC in Rathke cleft cysts were significantly higher than those in either the cystic components of craniopharyngiomas or the hemorrhagic components of pituitary adenomas, suggesting the use of DWI in differentiation of RCC from craniopharyngiomas (Kunii et al. 2007) (Fig. 3.4).
- *Astrocytomas* of the suprasellar region are usually intraparenchymal hypothalamic or chiasmatic masses. Calcifications and cysts are absent. Related to tumor grading, they do not enhance or may demonstrate peripheral enhancement (Fig. 3.5).
- *Pituitary adenoma*: this is a rare tumor in prepubertal children. The lesion is characteristically intrasellar with suprasellar growth. The tissue is more heterogeneous, with cystic, necrotic, and hemorrhagic components. Calcifications are absent (Hess and Dillon 2012; Choi et al. 2007) (Fig. 3.6).
- *Dermoid or epidermoid cyst*: they can be hyperintense on T1WI, related to fatty content, and may have calcifications. An *epidermoid cyst* (EC) is usually off-midline: suprasellar ECs are uncommon. Neither dermoid nor epidermoid cysts enhance. Epidermoid cysts shows high signal in DWI, while craniopharyngiomas don't (Pisaneschi and Kapoor 2005).
- *Germ cell tumors*: the lesion is typical of young-adult age, composed of a heterogeneous solid tissue with restricted diffusion. It may infiltrate the infundibulum and may seed within the surrounding subarachnoid space (Lee et al. 2014).
- *Aneurysms*: a giant aneurysm of distal carotid, with calcified walls, may mimic a craniopharyngioma – imaging features vary greatly depending on the grade of calcification and thrombosis present within the aneurysm. Contrast-enhanced CT may reveal an ovoidal parasagittal mass with homogeneous enhancement. There may be remodeling of the sella turcica. On MR imaging, a nonthrombosed aneurysm may appear as a rounded flow void that is contiguous with an adjacent arterial signal void. A thrombosed aneurysm may be heterogeneous both in MR signal intensity and CT density, because of the various stages of degradation hemoglobin (Pisaneschi and Kapoor 2005; Suh et al. 2001).

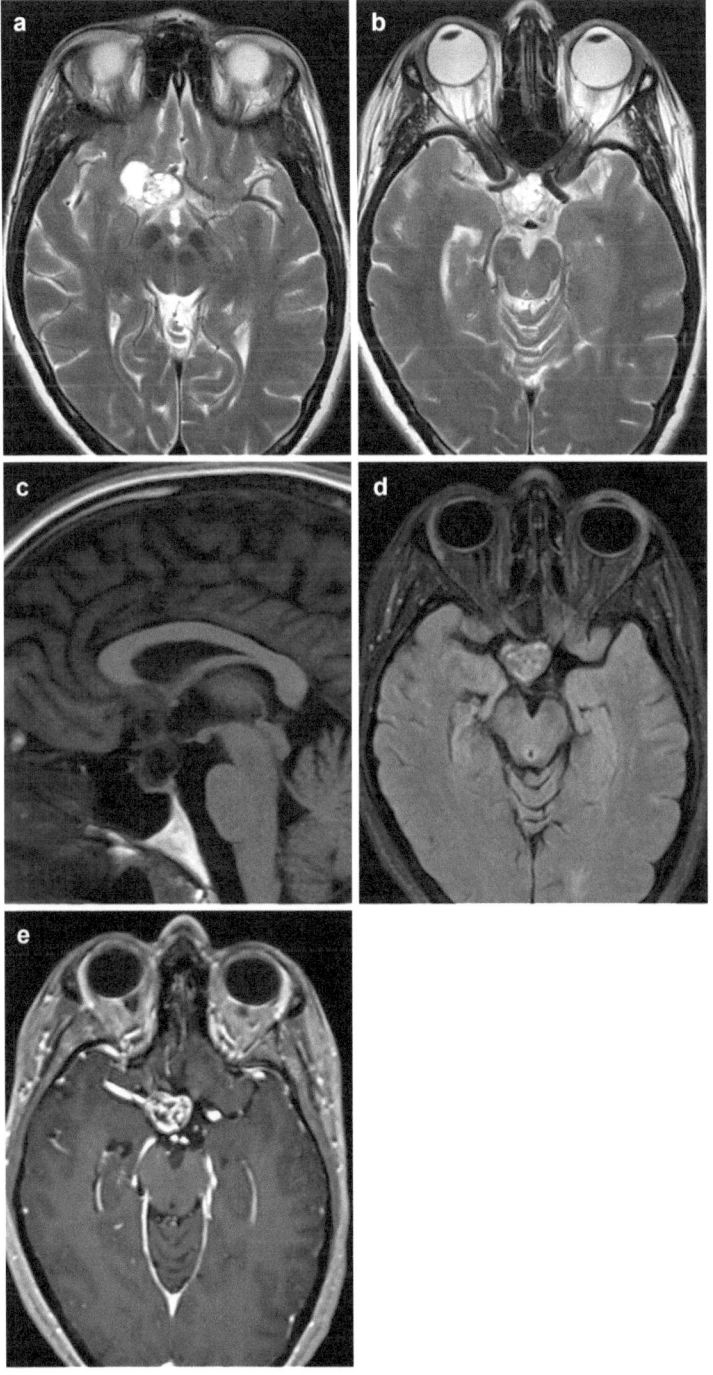

Fig. 3.3 Papillary craniopharyngioma. (**a**, **b**) Transverse T2WI demonstrates disomogeneous hyperintense suprasellar lesion, displacing the distal portion of carotid siphon and right middle cerebral artery origin; in (**c**), sagittal T1WI shows hypointense signal of the lesion, without any hyperintense spots. FLAIRWI (**d**) confirms the disomogeneous signal and the partial solid lesion. After administration of contrast media, marked, disomogeneous enhancement was noted on T1WI (**e**)

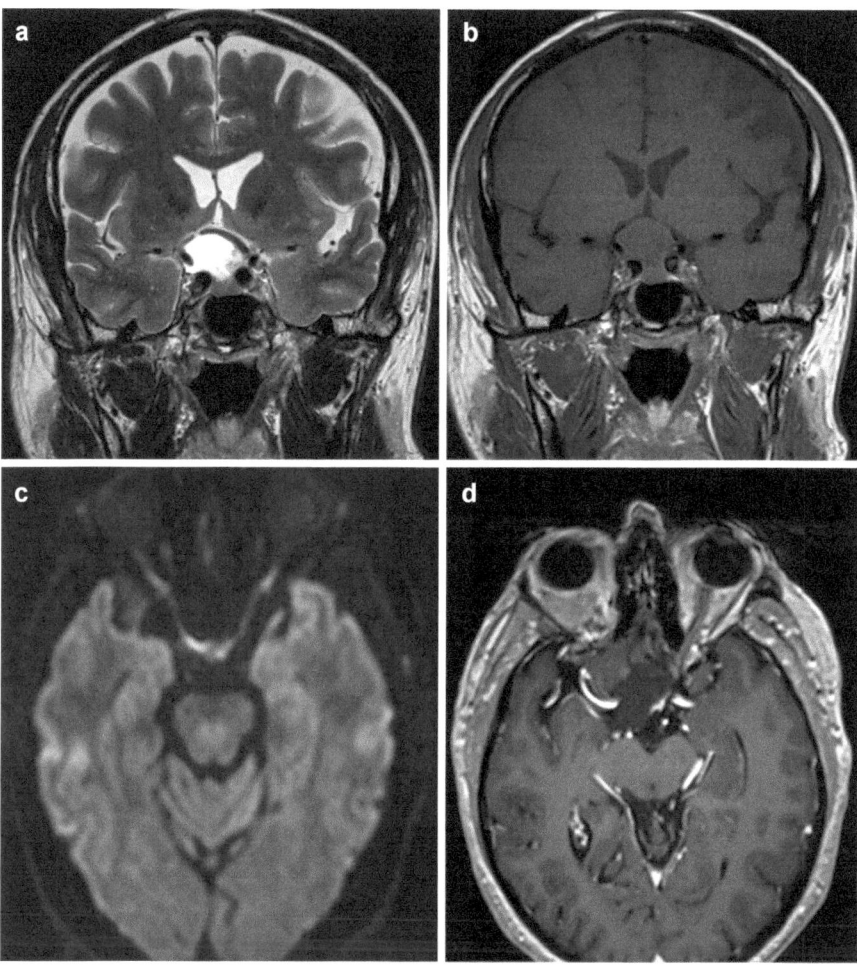

Fig. 3.4 Adamantinomatous craniopharyngioma. (**a**, **b**) Coronal T2WI and T1WI demonstrate hyperintense suprasellar/intrasellar lesion, with compression of optic chiasm and dislocation of right carotid siphon; in (**c**), no restricted diffusion on DWI. (**d**) After administration of contrast media, no enhancement on axial T1WI

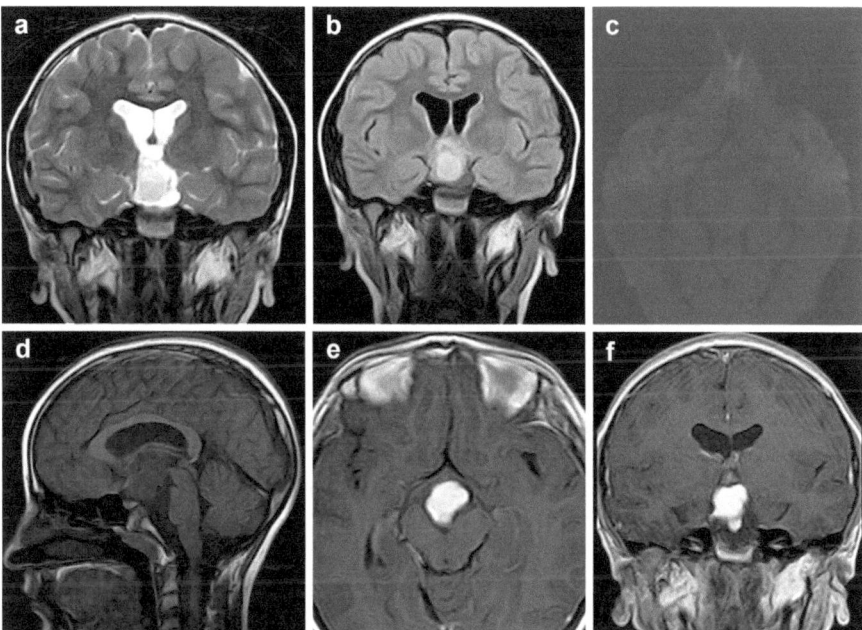

Fig. 3.5 Expansive suprasellar lesion, intra-axial. In (**a**), coronal T2WI demonstrates hyperintense tissue, confirmed at FLAIRWI (**b**), hypointense in T1WI (**d**). DWI (**c**) shows isointense signal to the brain. In (**e, f**), post-contrast T1WI, demonstrating homogeneous enhancement. Diagnosis: low-grade astrocytoma

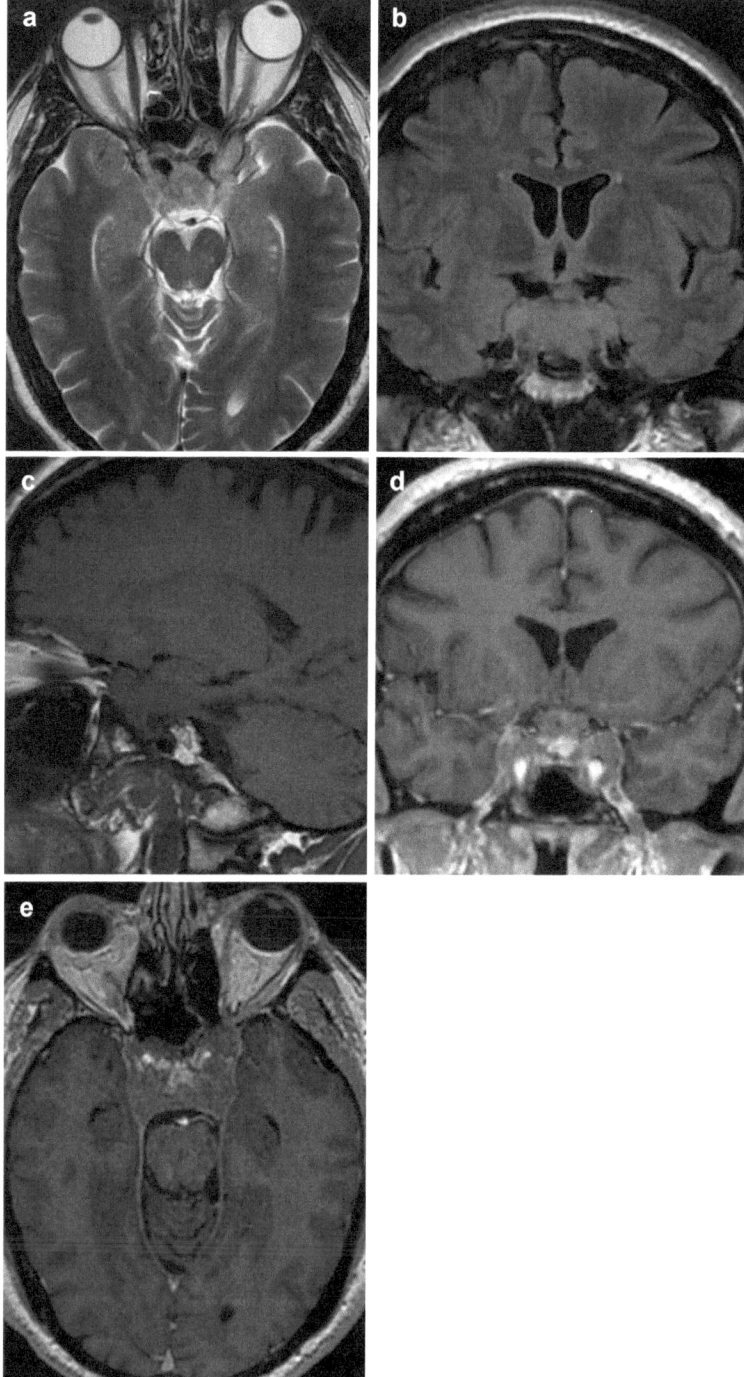

Fig. 3.6 Pituitary macroadenoma. (**a**) Transverse T2WI demonstrates disomogeneous intrasellar solid lesion, with invasion of both cavernous sinuses (best shown in (**b**, **c**), T1WI coronal and sagittal). After administration of gadolinium, partial disomogeneous enhancement was noted on T1WI (**d**, **e**)

Conclusion

Imaging is a nodal aspect in the diagnosis of craniopharyngioma: nowadays MRI is the gold standard for the detection of this suprasellar lesion, in addition to exploring its characteristics and relations to surrounding anatomical structures. CT is useful to detect intrinsic calcification, poorly detectable on MRI.

References

Ahmadi J et al (1992) Cystic fluid in craniopharyngiomas: MR imaging and quantitative analysis. Radiology 182(3):783–785

Borges A (2009) Imaging of the central skull base. Neuroimaging Clin N Am 19(4):669–696

Choi SH et al (2007) Pituitary adenoma, craniopharyngioma, and Rathke cleft cyst involving both intrasellar and suprasellar regions: differentiation using MRI. Clin Radiol 62(5):453–462

Crotty TB et al (1995) Papillary craniopharyngioma: a clinicopathological study of 48 cases. J Neurosurg 83(2):206–214

Curran JG, O'Connor E (2005) Imaging of craniopharyngioma. Childs Nerv Syst 21:635–639

Ginat DT, Meyers SP (2012) Intracranial lesions with high signal intensity on T1-weighted MR images: differential diagnosis. Radiographics 32(2):499–516

Hess CP, Dillon WP (2012) Imaging the pituitary and parasellar region. Neurosurg Clin N Am 23(4):529–542

Karavitaki N et al (2006) Craniopharyngiomas. Endocr Rev 27:371–397

Kunii N et al (2007) Rathke's cleft cysts: differentiation from other cystic lesions in the pituitary fossa by use of single-shot fast spin-echo diffusion-weighted MR imaging. Acta Neurochir 149(8):759–769

Lee H-J et al (2014) Pretreatment diagnosis of suprasellar papillary craniopharyngioma and germ cell tumors of adult patients. AJNR Am J Neuroradiol 36(3):508–517

Lucas JW, Zada G (2012) Imaging of the pituitary and parasellar region. Semin Neurol 32(4):320–331

Müller HL (2013) Childhood craniopharyngioma. Pituitary 16(1):56–67

Osborn AG, Preece MT (2006) Intracranial cysts: radiologic-pathologic correlation and imaging approach. Radiology 239(3):650–664

Osborn AG (2012) Osborn's Brain: Imaging, Pathology, and Anatomy – Amirsys, Salt Lake City, UT. ISBN 978-1-931884-21-1

Pisaneschi M, Kapoor G (2005) Imaging the sella and parasellar region. Neuroimaging Clin N Am 15:203–219

Prieto R, Pascual JM, Barrios L (2015) Optic chiasm distortions caused by craniopharyngiomas: clinical and magnetic resonance imaging correlation and influence on visual outcome. World Neurosurg 83(4):500–529

Sartoretti-Schefer S et al (1997) MR differentiation of adamantinous and squamous-papillary craniopharyngiomas. AJNR Am J Neuroradiol 18(1):77–87

Suh DC et al (2001) Supraclinoid internal carotid arterial aneurysm presenting as a suprasellar mass-like lesion in a child. Interv Neuroradiol 7(4):357–361

Tsuda M et al (1997) CT and MR imaging of craniopharyngioma. Eur Radiol 7(4):464–469

Van Effenterre R, Boch A-L (2002) Craniopharyngioma in adults and children: a study of 122 surgical cases. J Neurosurg 97(1):3–11

Weiner HL et al (1994) Craniopharyngiomas: a clinicopathological analysis of factors predictive of recurrence and functional outcome. Neurosurgery 35(6):1001–1011

Zada G et al (2010) Craniopharyngioma and other cystic epithelial lesions of the sellar region: a review of clinical, imaging, and histopathological relationships. Neurosurg Focus 28(4):E4

Timothy R. Smith, Breno Nery, Wenya Linda Bi,
Ian F. Dunn, and Edward R. Laws Jr.

Abstract

The surgical approach to craniopharyngioma (CP) treatment is complex. It is crucial to objectively define the advantages and limitations of each surgical option in terms of outcomes and risk of complications. The indications for and the success of transsphenoidal endoscopic approaches continue to expand, allowing for safe and efficient for tumor resection. Advancements in pre- and intraoperative imaging, microscopy, endoscopy, and refinements in medical management have all helped to improve patient outcomes for those harboring CPs. As the number and complexity of surgical tools increase, there is an increased need for attention to and consideration of the surgical approach itself. Not all approaches are appropriate for every CP, and the nuances of each individual case should guide the operative strategy.

4.1 Introduction

The initial description of a craniopharyngioma dates to over 150 years ago (Prabhu and Brown 2005; Zada et al. 2010). The first successful removal of a craniopharyngioma was performed transsphenoidally in 1909 by A. E. Halstead at Saint Luke's

T.R. Smith • B. Nery • W.L. Bi • I.F. Dunn
Department of Neurosurgery, Brigham and Women's Hospital, Harvard Medical School, Boston, MA, USA

E.R. Laws Jr., MD (✉)
Department of Neurosurgery, Harvard Medical School, Brigham and Women's Hospital, Boston, MA, USA

Dana-Faber Cancer Institute, Boston, MA, USA
e-mail: elaws@partners.org

© Springer International Publishing Switzerland 2016
A. Lania et al. (eds.), *Diagnosis and Management of Craniopharyngiomas: Key Current Topics*, DOI 10.1007/978-3-319-22297-4_4

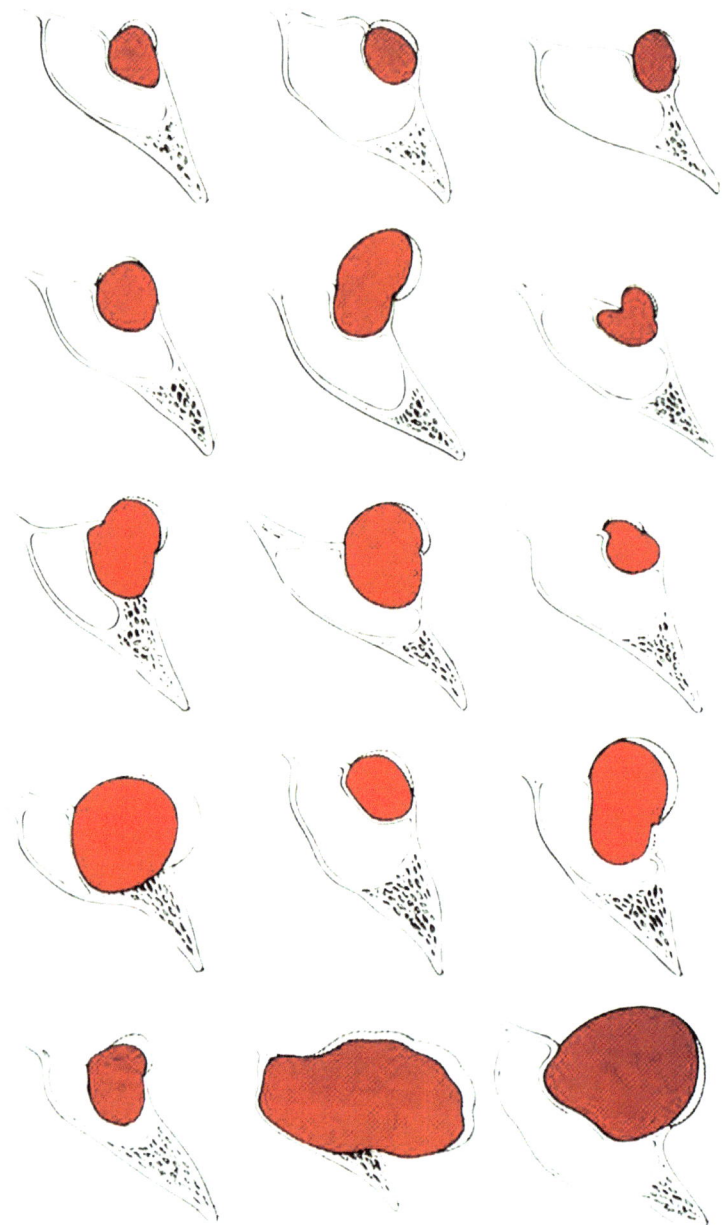

Fig. 4.1 Schematic illustrations of craniopharyngiomas operated through the transsphenoidal approach; sagittal view of the sella and sphenoid region with tumor depicted in auburn (From the collection of Dr. Edward Laws)

Hospital (Halstead 1910). Although craniopharyngiomas are considered histologically benign lesions, their anatomical location, physical characteristics, and biological behavior challenge their management (Fig. 4.1) (Elliott et al. 2011).

Fig. 4.2 Tuberoinfundibular embryologic origin of craniopharyngiomas, as represented by dots. More superior origins may result in suprasellar and third ventricular tumors, while inferiorly originating tumor nests along the infundibulum may result in an intrasellar craniopharyngioma (From the collection of Dr. Edward Laws)

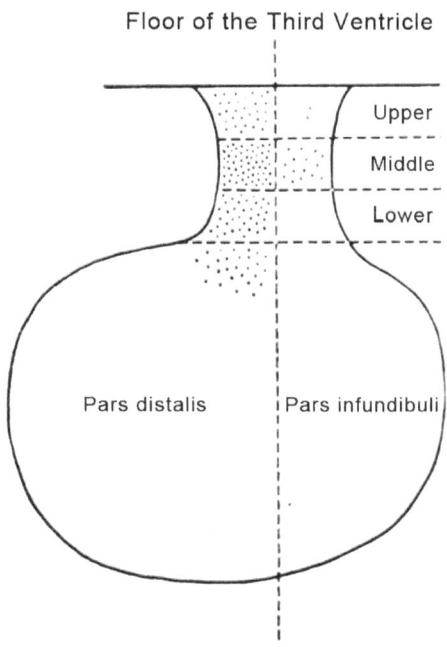

Floor of the Third Ventricle

Upper

Middle

Lower

Pars distalis   Pars infundibuli

Indeed, Harvey Cushing coined the term craniopharyngioma and deemed it "the most formidable of intracranial tumors" (Barkhoudarian and Laws 2013). Surgery continues to be at the heart of therapeutic strategies to manage these tumors. Initial complete surgical resection improves patient outcomes and overall survival and decreases recurrence risk across both pediatric and adult populations (Matson and Crigler 1969; Yasargil et al. 1990; Duff et al. 2000; Fahlbusch and Hofmann 2008). Gross total resection, however, is often challenging because of tumor adherence to surrounding structures, especially in cases of reoperation (Fahlbusch et al. 1999). Preservation of the pituitary stalk should be attempted whenever possible, unless panhypopituitarism and diabetes insipidus already exists and there is potential for total removal of a tumor originating within the infundibulum (Fig. 4.2). Conservative resection is warranted for tumors demonstrating invasion of the hypothalamus, as maintenance of high quality of life is a major priority (Zada et al. 2010). This chapter focuses on transsphenoidal approaches and adjuvant therapies.

4.2 Transsphenoidal Approaches

When craniopharyngiomas arise within the sella turcica, they usually compress, adhere to, and/or invade the pituitary gland and the infundibulum. For this reason, many patients present with hypopituitarism. If they do not have pituitary dysfunction prior to surgery, many will develop hypopituitarism following removal of an entirely intrasellar lesion. Transsphenoidal surgery is ideally suited as the primary approach for patients with evidence of pituitary dysfunction. When pituitary function is intact, usually with suprasellar lesions, it is sometimes easier to preserve function via a craniotomy (Oskouian et al. 2006). Until recently, transcranial approaches dominated for surgical management of craniopharyngiomas (Fahlbusch and Hofmann 2008; Fahlbusch et al. 1999; Laws 1987; Samii and Bini 1991). There are, however, an expanding number of patients in whom the transsphenoidal approach represents an alternative, if not superior, option (Cavallo et al. 2008; Fahlbusch and Hofmann 2008; Gardner et al. 2008a, b; Jane et al. 2010a, b; Komotar et al. 2009; Laws 1997; Maira et al. 2004; Teo 2005).

When considering a transsphenoidal approach to craniopharyngioma resection, the origin of the lesion with regard to the sella turcica and presence of any sellar enlargement should be understood (Fig. 4.2). When craniopharyngiomas originate above the diaphragm, the sella appears normal in size. Approximately one-third of craniopharyngiomas have their epicenter bellow the diaphragma sella (Honegger and Tatagiba 2008). In such cases, progressive enlargement of the sella can occur, an imaging feature seen in 30–60 % of cases of previously reported series (Horsley 1906; Komotar et al. 2012; Laws 1980). This is by far the most important consideration, because the advantage of this topography is that when the tumor grows, even if the dorsal tumor capsule fuses with the diaphragm, the craniopharyngioma does not extend through it. This prevents tumor attachment to neurovascular structures – in particular the optic chiasm, basal vasculature, and hypothalamus. An enlarged sella also permits greater room for surgery. For total removal of intrasellar craniopharyngiomas, it is often important to resect the diaphragm, as it is frequently inseparable from the tumor capsule (Laws 1997; Laws 1994).

Other critical anatomic features include the aeration and septation of the sphenoid sinus, the distance between the parasellar carotid arteries, and the relationship of the tumor to the infundibulum, the optic nerves and the chiasm, and vessels within the circle of Willis. Wider distance between the carotid arteries and enlargement of the sella makes intracranial manipulation more readily accomplished. The increasing integration of image guidance has contributed significantly to the safety and versatility of the endoscopic approach. The advent of expanded ventral skull base approaches and the operating endoscope has led to renewed enthusiasm regarding transsphenoidal management of craniopharyngiomas (Hochenegg 1908; Kaptain et al. 2001). Lesions with suprasellar, retroclinoidal, and posterior extension to the optic chiasm, even up to the third ventricle, are excellent candidates for the transsphenoidal approach, because of the parallel trajectory between the growth of craniopharyngiomas and the endoscopic surgical axis. With the introduction of 3D intraoperative endoscopic technology, previous challenges with depth perception are ameliorated.

Transsphenoidal approaches for craniopharyngiomas have been associated with increased gross total resection, decreased recurrence, and lower incidence of hypothalamic obesity and permanent diabetes insipidus when compared to transcranial approaches (Jane et al. 2010a, b; Komotar et al. 2012). Endonasal approaches may also lead to comparable or even improved visual outcomes compared to open transcranial approaches (Fahlbusch et al. 1999; Komotar et al. 2012). Craniotomy, however, may be superior in craniopharyngiomas with extensive calcification, involvement of circle of Willis vasculature, eccentric location with lateral extension to the cavernous sinus, and adherence to the hypothalamus (Elliott et al. 2011; Giordano 1897).

4.2.1 Microscopic Transsphenoidal Approaches

4.2.1.1 Sublabial

Today, the sublabial transsphenoidal approach is sometimes employed in pediatric cases, secondary to the relatively small nares in children. Some authors favor this approach because it provides a slightly less oblique orientation to the sella, a larger retractor width, and increased speculum stability. The wide exposure of the sella reveals the medial aspect of the anterior face of the bilateral cavernous sinuses, tuberculum sellae, and sellar floor within the same field of view under the operating microscope. We believe that these advantages can also be achieved with endonasal endoscopic approaches, with excellent exposure of all the structures mentioned above.

4.2.1.2 Endonasal

For transnasal and endonasal approaches, the initial opening varies from a superficial transcolumellar incision, a hemi-transfixion incision immediately posterior to the columella, and an incision at the junction of the bony and cartilaginous septum or at the junction of the bony nasal septum with the sphenoid rostrum (Griffith and Veerapen 1987; Kern et al. 1979; Kim et al. 2011; Wilson et al. 1990).

4.2.2 Transsphenoidal Transsellar Transdiaphragmatic Approach

Historically, this approach was utilized for craniopharyngiomas with intrasellar components and suprasellar extension. Usually, while undertaking the transsphenoidal resection of a sellar lesion, an intracapsular approach is preferred, when possible, to avoid complications resulting from the disruption of the diaphragma sella or from entering the cavernous sinus. In the transsphenoidal transsellar transdiaphragmatic approach, once the sellar portion of the tumor has been removed, the suprasellar component is excised by transgressing the tumor capsule and diaphragma to enter the subarachnoid space. The diaphragma is often inseparable from a craniopharyngioma and often needs to be excised in order to obtain a complete resection, deliberately creating a large CSF fistula.

4.2.3 Transsphenoidal Transtuberculum Sellae Approach

Frequently, craniopharyngiomas are situated in the suprasellar cistern in relation to the pituitary stalk. In 1987, Weiss described an innovative technique for accessing purely suprasellar tumors (Weiss 1987). This variation or "extension" of the transsphenoidal approach facilitates access to such lesions by a more rostral approach with removal of the tuberculum sellae and the planum sphenoidale. The underlying dura is then widely opened after careful ligation and division of the intercavernous sinus. This exposes the chiasmal cistern and permits a supradiaphragmatic view of the contents of the basal cisterns.

4.2.3.1 Cystic Suprasellar Craniopharyngiomas

Transsphenoidal drainage of large, predominantly cystic craniopharyngiomas is a useful strategy (Fig. 4.3). This is particularly helpful to alleviate symptomatic pressure on the optic chiasm. It is also useful following multiple redo procedures, in the presence of hydrocephalus from obstruction of the foramina of Monro, as a palliative procedure, or as a precursor to transcranial resection of the more solid component or capsule of the tumor – allowing it to retract from the hypothalamus (von Eiselsberg 1907). This approach allows the aspiration and drainage of a tumor cyst under direct vision. Drainage of a large suprasellar cystic component often results in mobilization of the tumor capsule into the operative field (Cushing 1909). On the other hand, tumors with a solid suprasellar component are unlikely to descend to within reach of resection of a conventional transsphenoidal approach. Heavily calcified tumors are even more resistant to mobilization.

4.2.3.2 Endoscopic Endonasal

The introduction of the endoscope, either as an adjunct to the microsurgical approach or as in isolation, has extended the scope of transsphenoidal procedures (Cappabianca et al. 2002; Jho 1997). The endoscope, pioneered by Gerard Guiot in the 1960s (Guiot et al. 1959), offers the major advantage of panoramic views, allowing identification of structures in the lateral walls of the sphenoid sinus and thereby

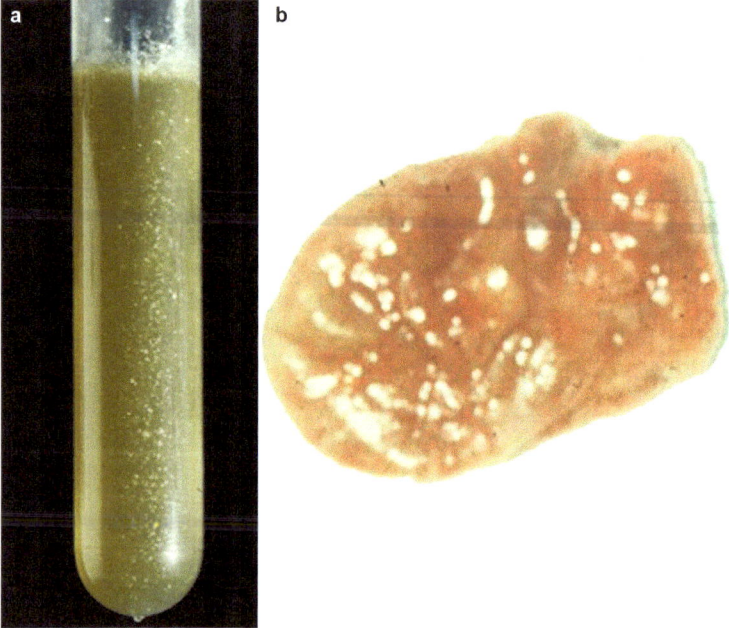

Fig. 4.3 (**a**) Intratumoral cystic content and (**b**) tumor capsule from a craniopharyngioma resected transsphenoidally (From the collection of Dr. Edward Laws)

maximizing exposure. It further provides angled views, facilitating resection under direct vision of suprasellar and lateral extensions of tumors, albeit at the expense of some loss of depth perception.

4.2.4 Anterior Skull Base Endoscopic Approach

Anterior skull base approaches take advantage of the surgical anatomy of the patient and the lesion and include microscopic endoscope-assisted and purely endoscopic techniques (Couldwell et al. 2004; Cavallo et al. 2009; de Divitiis 2013; Divitiis et al. 2007a, b; Dusick et al. 2005; Frank et al. 2006; Gardner et al. 2008a, b; Kim et al. 2011; Leng et al. 2012). Resection of the base of the sella, the tuberculum sellae, and the planum sphenoidale provides excellent access along the long axis of the craniopharyngioma, recognizing that if the tumor is retrochiasmatic, then it is intimately associated with the hypothalamus. Early experience with anterior skull base endoscopic approaches evolved in attempt to achieve gross total removal of craniopharyngiomas (Kaptain et al. 2001). The development of modern microsurgical instrumentation, finely controlled drills, frameless stereotaxy, microvascular Doppler ultrasound, the operating microscope, precision ultrasonic aspirator, and the endoscope has extended its role even further (Couldwell et al. 2004).

This approach offers several advantages. Its main advantage is that midline exposure is achieved without brain retraction, enabling face-on exposure of the tumor. The exposure provided is often wider than that achieved by frontotemporal and subfrontal approaches. It has the added advantage of exposing the tumor-brain interface under direct vision, not around blind corners. It circumvents need for an enlarged sella and is not as restricted by the position of the chiasm as in a transcranial approach. It also facilitates rapid debulking of the tumor, enabling mobilization of the tumor capsule. Transsphenoidal anterior skull base approaches are also associated with greater risk of CSF leak, bleeding, and need for a septal flap.

When craniopharyngiomas are situated exclusively in the suprasellar cistern in relation to the pituitary stalk, the transsphenoidal transtuberculum sellae approach is a good option for tumor resection. Removal of the tuberculum sellae and the planum sphenoidale permits exposure of the chiasmatic cistern and a supradiaphragmatic view of the contents of the basal cisterns (Cushing 1909; Weiss 1987).

4.2.5 Combined Approaches

The optimal surgical management strategy for complex craniopharyngiomas may involve a combination of transcranial and transsphenoidal approaches, either simultaneously or in separate sittings. The introduction of extended transsphenoidal approaches and endoscopic approaches has reduced the frequency with which combined approaches are used.

4.3   Endonasal Transsphenoidal Operative Technique

The endonasal transseptal transsphenoidal approach has been applied with superb results for craniopharyngiomas (Laws and Jane 2010). Preoperative preparation, operative setup, and surgical technique will be reviewed.

4.3.1   Preoperative Phase

Any history of prior nasal surgery should be documented, as it can influence the surgical approach. Imaging review is a mainstay in preoperative evaluation (Fig. 4.4). The paranasal sinuses are inspected for deviated septum and septal bony spurs, which may impact the nasal phase of the operation. The pneumatization of the

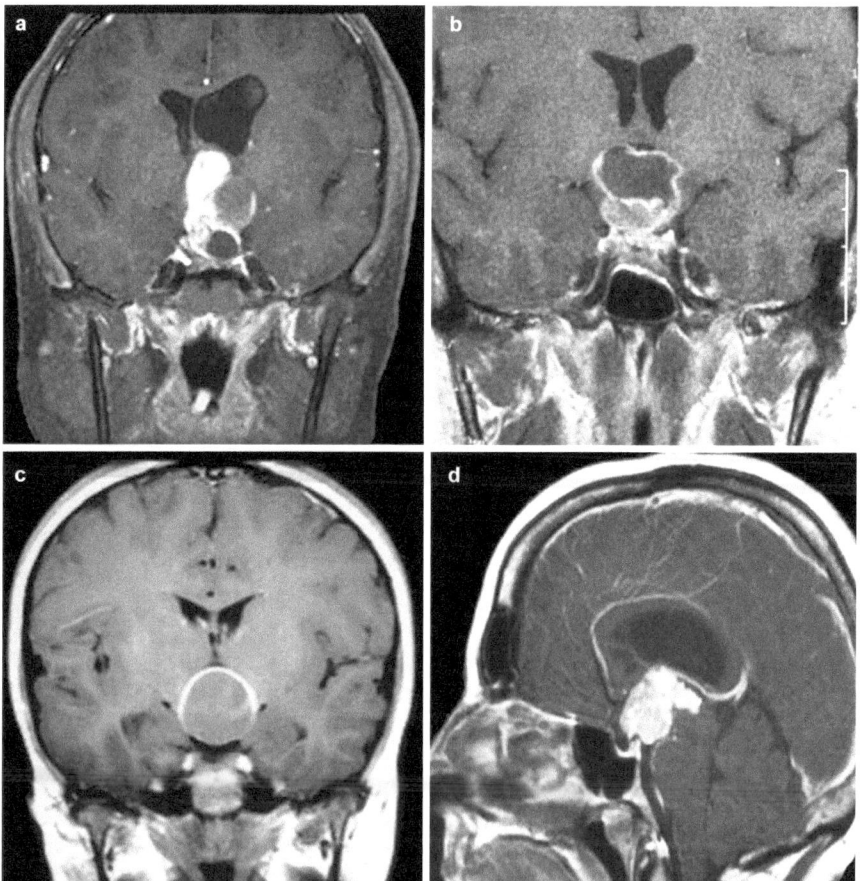

Fig. 4.4 MRI of craniopharyngiomas. T1-weighted gadolinium-enhanced MRI in (**a–c**) coronal and (**d**) sagittal view

sphenoid is noted (conchal, pre-sellar, sellar), to help plan the degree of drilling needed to expose the sella, often under neuronavigation guidance (Zada et al. 2011). The sphenoid sinus is inspected for thin septae, which are often off midline and frequently lead towards an internal carotid artery. These are important landmarks for the sphenoidal phase of the operation. The contour of the sellar face is noted and as is its relationship to the planum sphenoidale and clivus. The suprasellar cistern is evaluated, noting the position of the optic chiasm, stalk, and anterior cerebral arteries relative to the lesion. The surgeon should have a clear understanding of the location of the normal pituitary gland prior to beginning the sellar phase. A preoperative endocrine evaluation should be complete. Perioperative steroids are typically administered prior to incision when appropriate. Patients with a preoperative fasting cortisol less than 10 mcg/dL receive preoperative and intraoperative stress doses. Nasal prep begins in the preoperative care unit with oxymetazoline solution 0.05 % (Afrin™) applied to each nostril every 15 min.

4.3.2 Operating Room Layout and Patient Positioning

The patient table is rotated approximately 170° from anesthesia, such that when the patient's head is tilted towards the left shoulder, the midline of the head parallels the walls of the room, and the dorsum of the nose parallels the floor. For significant intracranial involvement, some extension of the head is helpful. The table is positioned in reflex with torso elevated 15–20°, and the legs down, approximating a beach chair. The ultimate goal of positioning is to aim the patient's nares directly at the surgeon when the surgeon is standing at the right arm, with the head elevated sufficiently above the heart to minimize venous congestion. Some extension of the head may be appropriate in extended cases where drilling of the tuberculum sella and the planum sphenoidale is anticipated. The right arm is tucked, and the left arm is placed on an arm board for anesthesia to have access. Once positioned, the operative bed can be adjusted up, down, or reverse Trendelenburg. Any other movements risk traction on the neck if the head is fixed in pins. Neuronavigation is registered if being used.

An orogastric tube (OGT) is placed prior to surgery, to allow evacuation of swallowed blood from the stomach following the operation and help prevent postoperative nausea/vomiting. Endotracheal tubes are secured to the left side of the mouth, with tape along the lower lip and jaw only. A bite block is placed. After intubation, the nares are swabbed with aqueous antibiotic-soaked cotton applicators, followed by packing with cottonoid strips soaked in oxymetazoline (0.05 % solution). After the table is rotated to the desired surgical position, the oxymetazoline-soaked cottonoid patties are swapped for patties soaked in 1 % lidocaine with 1:100,000 epinephrine. The abdomen is prepared for a fat graft. We typically use a subumbilical ("smile") incision – 2 to 3 cm buried in the skin fold of the umbilicus – unless the patient has had prior abdominal surgery. This is prepped with betadine or a similar antiseptic solution. The eyes are protected with occlusive dressing. Skin adhesive is placed across the bridge of the nose and the upper lip to help the towels adhere when draping the nose. We strongly recommend performing an operative checklist after draping to confirm that there are no unanticipated operative issues, that anesthesia has delivered antibiotics within 60 min of starting, that corticosteroids have been given when indicated, and that no dexamethasone is administered for nausea prophylaxis.

4.3.3 Surgical Procedure

4.3.3.1 Nasal Phase (Single Surgeon/Two Hands)

The nasal phase begins with the introduction of a short 0° 18 cm endoscope in the right nostril. After the floor of the nasal cavity and inferior turbinates are identified, the endoscope and a 9 Fr suction are advanced to identify the choana and aspirate any secretions. The inferior turbinate is identified and lateralized. The middle turbinate is lateralized from inferior to superior, to prevent injury to the mucosa. As the superior turbinate is identified, it is compressed laterally in the same manner, avoiding undue pressure on its vertical lamella, which can be transmitted to and fracture the cribriform plate. This usually exposes the sphenoid ostium, located 1.5 cm above the arch of the choana. The septal mucosa is infiltrated with local anesthetic, especially along the junction of the perpendicular plate with the septal cartilage where the septal mucosal incision is made. The mucosa overlying the vomer to the approximate location of the sphenopalatine trunk is also infiltrated. The nostril is packed with cottonoid patties soaked in lidocaine, and this procedure is performed following the same steps in the left nostril.

Following infiltration with local anesthetic, the ostium is again identified, and the mucosa surrounding it is cauterized. The ostium is enlarged on each side, primarily on its medial and superior borders, taking care with the inferolateral border, where septal branches of the sphenopalatine artery cross the vomer. Once the ostium is enlarged, the sphenoid sinus and its mucosa are visualized along with the bulge of the sella itself. Next, the junction of the bony and cartilaginous septum is identified at the anterior edge of the middle turbinate, and a vertical mucosal incision is made at this junction. A subperichondral tunnel is fashioned in a craniocaudal fashion, and the junction of ethmoidal perpendicular plate, vomer, and sphenoid rostrum is visualized. The mucosa is dissected away from the sphenoid rostrum, exposing the contralateral sphenoid ostium. Posterior portions of the bony nasal septum (perpendicular plate) are removed with pituitary rongeurs, and the mobilized septal mucosa is reflected or resected with a microdebrider. This maneuver completes the posterior septectomy, which allows a binasal approach. The sphenoidotomy is performed with Kerrison rongeurs, extending from the planum sphenoidale superiorly to the floor of the sphenoid inferiorly and laterally to expose the carotid protuberances. Sphenoid septations can be removed with a rongeur or drill, creating unimpeded access to the sella for the endoscope and instruments. Anatomical landmarks are confirmed with neuronavigation prior to and after the sphenoidal phase. Rarely, turbinates may be resected if extra room is needed.

4.3.3.2 Sphenoidal Phase (Two Surgeons, Three or Four Hands)

The sphenoidal phase begins with the assistant (standing alongside the head) introducing a long 0° 30 cm endoscope into the right nostril. The primary surgeon introduces all instruments underneath the 0° endoscope. After the sphenoid mucosa is reflected or removed over the sellar bone, the face of the sella is opened without violation of the sella dura. There is often a dehiscence through which a blunt nerve hook can be introduced to develop the epidural plane where the sellar bone is attenuated. A Kerrison punch or diamond drill follows, exposing sellar dura from the edge of the tuberculum to the floor of the sella, and cavernous sinus to cavernous sinus laterally. The microvascular Doppler is used to identify the cavernous carotid arteries, demarcating the lateral margins of the exposure.

4.3.3.3 Sellar Phase

The dura is incised to minimize damage to the underlying pituitary capsule. In the case of craniopharyngiomas, an "H"-shaped incision is often chosen to create a subdural dissection plane between the tumor capsule and the pituitary gland. The superior intercavernous sinus lies beneath the tuberculum and is often a robust structure that presents a barrier to the requisite exposure. Prior to dividing the superior intercavernous sinus, it should be occluded by electrocautery, hemostatic agents, and/or occasionally with hemostatic clips. The dura can then be opened like a book and provides excellent exposure of the arachnoid membrane above the floor of the frontal fossa and above the sellar diaphragm.

This initial exposure allows dissection and/or mobilization of the residual pituitary gland in the floor of the sella. The decision to mobilize or resect the gland is dependent of the patient's preoperative endocrine status. When the patient has panhypopituitarism (including diabetes insipidus), the superior aspect of the pituitary gland can be dissected to the insertion of the stalk. Sharp dissection of the pituitary stalk liberates the inferior aspect of the tumor from its attachments to the sella. Subsequent to this, it is necessary to detach the remnant of the diaphragm of the sella from its attachments to the tuberculum anteriorly and to the dorsum sellae and posterior clinoids posteriorly. In tumors that arise within the sella, the diaphragm acts as a barrier between the superior aspect of the tumor, optic chiasm, and hypothalamus, and its resection aids in obtaining complete removal.

The arachnoid is carefully opened to expose the anterior face of the tumor. Maintaining the arachnoid plane is the initial goal. After initial debulking of the lesion, the tumor is separated from the inferior aspect of the optic chiasm, with careful preservation of chiasmatic microvasculature supply. Once this is accomplished, further debulking of the lesion ultimately allows mobilization of the inferolateral aspects of the tumor, mobilization from the vessels of the circle of Willis, and ultimately from its attachments to the hypothalamus. These manipulations are accomplished using the operating endoscope, a variety of suctions, and micro-instruments, including cupped forceps and dissectors. After significant tumor removal, 30° angle endoscopes can be useful to extend lines of sight laterally, inferiorly, and superiorly. Long bipolar instruments are essential for the coagulation of capsular vessels. These vessels must be controlled in a methodical and progressive fashion in order to prevent hemorrhage from the dorsal aspect of the tumor.

The most difficult aspect of the operation is dissection of the tumor away from the hypothalamus. Frequently, there is a gliotic border that can be identified and carefully separated from the capsule of the tumor. Unfortunately, there is often invasion of the brain in this area by the tumor itself, and overly aggressive resection can result in devastating damage to the hypothalamus producing both memory loss and hypothalamic obesity (Page-Wilson et al. 2012; Hamilton et al. 2011). For this reason, it sometimes becomes necessary to leave tumor remnants attached to the area of the hypothalamus, which are then treated by adjunctive radiosurgery or radiotherapy. Inspection is carried out with a 0° and/or 30° endoscope in systematic fashion – inferior, posterior, cavernous sinus walls, and finally the diaphragma sellae, inspecting for any residual tumor or hemorrhagic source.

4.3.4 Closure

Once the tumor is removed to the greatest and safest extent possible, closure becomes a major challenge. The intentional disruption of the integrity of the subarachnoid space is contrary to customary practice of transsphenoidal surgery and magnifies the potential for postoperative CSF rhinorrhea and meningitis.

Initial attempts using the extended transsphenoidal approach had postoperative CSF leak rates ranging from 10 to 58 % (Couldwell et al. 2004; Dedivitiis et al. 2007a, b; Dusick et al. 2005, 2008; Gardner et al. 2008a, b; Kaptain et al. 2001; Weiss 1987). A number of solutions have been proposed with various methods of reconstructing the skull base, and each has a certain advantages. The advent of the vascularized nasal septal flap repair of the face of the sella has revolutionized this aspect of the operation, and subsequent CSF leakage has decreased to 4–5 % (Kassam et al. 2008; Hadad et al. 2006). The incidence of these complications ranges from 2 to 6.5 % for CSF leak and 0.4–2 % for meningitis in transsphenoidal series where extracapsular resection is not an objective of surgery (Shapiro et al. 1979).

After tumor resection and hemostasis, the tumor cavity is gently packed with an abdominal fat graft. This should be of sufficient quantity to fill the dead space, but not so much as to create a mass lesion. A gasket seal closure using fascia lata buttressed by a Medpor plate or a stent of nasal bone or cartilage is fashioned and placed epidurally to reconstruct the sellar floor. The vascularized mucosal flap is placed over the sellar opening and can be reinforced by a fat graft placed within the sphenoid sinus, with or without tissue glue. After meticulous hemostasis within the nasal passages, evacuation of excess fluid/blood in the nasopharynx, and medialization of the turbinates, lubricated nasal packs are placed bilaterally when needed. These packs are typically removed 1–2 days after the operative procedure while the patient is still in the hospital, depending on the extent of intraoperative CSF leak.

4.4 Adjuvant Therapy

4.4.1 Intracavitary Radioisotopes

The majority of craniopharyngiomas have cystic components (Spaziante et al. 1989; Young et al. 1987; Zona and Spaziante 2006), which results in the clinical symptoms. When cystic pathology is the predominant feature of a craniopharyngioma, intracavitary radiation can lead to cessation of cyst fluid accumulation and gradual cyst shrinkage. Leksell and Liden first reported on the use of intracavitary therapy for cystic craniopharyngiomas with the colloidal, purely beta-emitting radioisotope phosphorus-32 (^{32}P) in 1952 (Leksell 1952). Since that time, other isotopes have been utilized including ^{90}Y (Huk and Mahlstedt 1983; Szeifert et al. 1990; Blackburn et al. 1999) and ^{186}Re (Derrey et al. 2008). The most recent reports of cyst control using these isotopes range from 63 to 100 %, with stable to improved vision in 50–94 % (Barriger et al. 2011; Derrey et al. 2008; Hasegawa et al. 2004; Julow et al. 2007; Kickingereder et al. 2012; Van den berger et al. 1992).

4.4.2 Intracavitary Chemotherapy

Bleomycin is a chemotherapeutic agent used against epithelial tumors (Mottolese et al. 2001). It was thought to be useful in selected cases of predominantly cystic craniopharyngiomas, especially cystic recurrence in young children where radiotherapy should be delayed or avoided. Recent experience with longer follow-up has shown that although the response rate is initially high, the rate of regression free survival is poor (Caceres 2005; Laws et al. 2003). Bleomycin therapy is furthermore associated with serious complications related to its toxicity and hypothalamic damage following instillation after subtotal resection, ischemic attacks, peritumoral edema, cranial nerve palsies, blindness, and death related to drug migration into the CSF space (Hader et al. 2000; Liu et al. 2012; Mottolese et al. 2001).

4.4.3 Interferon Therapy

Craniopharyngiomas originate from the same progenitor cells as squamous cell skin carcinoma, which can be treated successfully with interferon-alpha (IFNα)-2a. Patients with progressive or recurrent craniopharyngiomas have been treated with systemic IFNα. In particular, 50 % of patients with cyst-predominant craniopharyngiomas had a complete response after receiving intracystic administration of IFNα-2a. In a prospective multicenter study of 60 pediatric patients, Cavalheiro et al. evaluated the efficacy of intratumoral INFα-based chemotherapy. Clinical and radiological improvement was reported in 76 % of patients along with new endocrinologic deficits in 13 % of patients. Interferon therapy holds promise as part of the panoply of therapeutic strategies for craniopharyngioma treatment.

4.5 Outcomes

Patients with craniopharyngioma are "managed" as opposed to "cured." Survival rates are favorable, but recurrence must be anticipated. Long-term survival rates approach 93 % at 10 years following radical surgical resection of craniopharyngiomas (Fahlbusch et al. 1999). Long-term recurrence-free survival rates are variable, have been reported as approximately 38–87 % at 10 years postoperatively, and depend largely on the extent of tumor resection (Fahlbusch et al. 1999; Karavitaki et al. 2005). Reported gross total resection rates vary from 45 to 90 %, depending on the approach and tumor characteristics reported (Fahlbusch et al. 1999; Chakrabarti et al. 2005; Yasargil et a.1990). Gross total resection is far less likely for recurrent craniopharyngiomas as compared to de novo tumors (Laws 1980). On review of the literature, the spectra of 5- and 10-year survival rates were 58–100 % and 24–100 % for total resection, 37–71 % and 31–52 % for subtotal excision, and 69–95 % and 62–84 % for subtotal resection and postoperative radiotherapy (Elliott et al. 2011).

The subtype of craniopharyngioma, adamantinomatous or papillary, also influences the extent of resection, recurrence rate, and overall outcome (Yasargil et al. 1990). In general, adamantinomatous craniopharyngiomas demonstrate a higher potential for recurrence than the squamous-papillary subtype (Yasargil et al. 1990; Weiner et al. 1994; Crotty et al. 1995; Adamson et al. 1990). They may also carry a poorer outcome (Adamson et al. 1990), possibly related to their propensity for the pediatric population.

Visual improvement is noted in 74–87 % of craniopharyngioma patients following surgery, with greater improvement noted following transsphenoidal surgery than transcranial approaches (Chakrabarti et al. 2005; Kim et al. 2011; Laws 1980; Leng et al. 2012; Yamada et al. 2010). Some degree of hypopituitarism requiring hormonal replacement therapy is required in 65–90 % of patients (Honegger et al. 1999), and panhypopituitarism occurs in up to 43 % of patients following surgery (Honegger et al. 1999). Permanent DI develops in up to 60 % of cases postoperatively (Honegger et al. 1999).

CSF leak has been reported to in 1.5–17 % of cases following craniopharyngioma operations (Maira et al. 1995; Maira et al. 2004; Laws 1994; Kim et al. 2011; Fahlbusch et al. 1999; Dusick et al. 2005; Chakrabarti et al. 2005). Meningitis and mortality are infrequent occurrences across modern surgical series for craniopharyngiomas.

Long-term cardiovascular, neurological, and psychosocial morbidities can reach 22 %, 49 %, and 47 %, respectively. The complication of a hypothalamic syndrome with affective disturbances postoperatively associated with obesity and psychosocial deterioration is both devastating and refractory to management with appetite suppressants. Recently, laparoscopic gastric banding has shown some promise as a treatment modality in postoperative morbid obesity (Muller et al. 2007).

Craniopharyngiomas are associated with excessive long-term multisystem morbidity and mortality, and this is especially true in female patients. The purpose of the follow-up should be to screen for recurrence and to ensure appropriate endocrine replacement. This is particularly important with respect to growth hormone replacement in children and estrogen replacement in premenopausal females. It is also important to manage glucose levels, lipids, blood pressure, and weight, as patients with craniopharyngiomas are at increased risk for cardiovascular disease. Despite intensive multimodal treatment, high rates of endocrinopathy, and the possibility of recurrence, patients do report a satisfactory quality of life after surgery (Laffond et al. 2012). In particular, endoscopic approaches are showing promise with regard to improved quality of life.

Conclusion

In dealing with craniopharyngiomas, it is crucial to objectively define the advantages and limits of each surgical technique in terms of outcomes and the prevention of complications. The indications and success of transsphenoidal endoscopic approaches continue to expand, allowing for safe and efficient for tumor resection. Video imaging (high definition and 3D visualization) is now a reality that has improved this surgical field, allowing the endoscope to offer good depth perception. Bimanual microsurgical technique as applied to endoscopic approaches overcomes limitations in tactile feedback. Ultimately, equipoise in assessing each case individually will dictate the optimal outcome (Zada and Cappabianca 2010).

References

Adamson TE, Wiestler OD, Kleihues P et al (1990) Correlation of clinical and pathological features in surgically treated craniopharyngiomas. J Neurosurg 73:12–17

Barkhoudarian G, Laws ER (2013) Craniopharyngioma: history. Pituitary 16:1–8

Barriger RB, Chang A, Lo SS et al (2011) Phosphorus-32 therapy for cystic craniopharyngiomas. Radiother Oncol 98:207–212

Blackburn TP, Doughty D, Plowman PN (1999) Stereotactic intracavitary therapy of recurrent cystic craniopharyngioma by instillation of 90yttrium. Br J Neurosurg 13:359–365

Caceres A (2005) Intracavitary therapeutic options in the management of cystic craniopharyngioma. Childs Nerv Syst 21:705–718

Cappabianca PCL, Colao AM, de Divitiis E (2002) Surgical complications associated with the endoscopic endonasal transsphenoidal approach for pituitary adenomas. J Neurosurg 97:293–298

Cavallo LM, Prevedello D, Esposito F et al (2008) The role of the endoscope in the transsphenoidal management of cystic lesions of the sellar region. Neurosurg Rev 31:55–64; discussion 64

Cavallo LM, Prevedello DM, Solari D et al (2009) Extended endoscopic endonasal transsphenoidal approach for residual or recurrent craniopharyngiomas. J Neurosurg 111:578–589

Chakrabarti I, Amar AP, Couldwell W et al (2005) Long-term neurological, visual, and endocrine outcomes following transnasal resection of craniopharyngioma. J Neurosurg 102:650–657

Couldwell WT, Weiss MH, Rabb C et al (2004) Variations on the standard transsphenoidal approach to the sellar region, with emphasis on the extended approaches and parasellar approaches: surgical experience in 105 cases. Neurosurgery 55:539–547

Crotty TB, Scheithauer BW, Young WF et al (1995) Papillary craniopharyngioma: a clinicopathological study of 48 cases. J Neurosurg 83:206–214

Cushing H (1909) Partial hypophysectomy for acromegaly: with remarks on the function of the hypophysis. Ann Surg 50:1002

de Divitiis E (2013) Endoscopic endonasal transsphenoidal surgery: from the pituitary fossa to the midline cranial base. World Neurosurg 80:e45–e51 de Divitiis E, Cappabianca P, Cavallo LM et al (2007a) Extended endoscopic transsphenoidal approach for extrasellar craniopharyngiomas. Neurosurgery 61:219–227

de Divitiis E, Cavallo LM, Cappabianca P et al (2007b) Extended endoscopic endonasal transsphenoidal approach for the removal of suprasellar tumors: Part 2. Neurosurgery 60: 46–58; discussion 58–49

Derrey S, Blond S, Reyns N et al (2008) Management of cystic craniopharyngiomas with stereotactic endocavitary irradiation using colloidal 186Re: a retrospective study of 48 consecutive patients. Neurosurgery 63:1045–1052

Duff J, Meyer FB, Ilstrup DM, Laws ER Jr, Schleck CD, Scheithauer BW (2000) Long-term outcomes for surgically resected craniopharyngiomas. Neurosurgery 46:291–302; discussion 302–395

Dusick JR, Esposito F, Kelly DF et al (2005) The extended direct endonasal transsphenoidal approach for nonadenomatous suprasellar tumors. J Neurosurg 102:832–841

Dusick JR, Fatemi N, Mattozo C et al (2008) Pituitary function after endonasal surgery for nonadenomatous parasellar tumors: Rathke's cleft cysts, craniopharyngiomas, and meningiomas. Surg Neurol 70:482–490

Elliott RE, Jane JA Jr, Wisoff JH (2011) Surgical management of craniopharyngiomas in children: meta-analysis and comparison of transcranial and transsphenoidal approaches. Neurosurgery 69:630–643

Fahlbusch R, Hofmann BM (2008) Surgical management of giant craniopharyngiomas. Acta Neurochir 150:1213–1226

Fahlbusch R, Honegger J, Paulus W et al (1999) Surgical treatment of craniopharyngiomas: experience with 168 patients. J Neurosurg 90:237–250

Frank G, Pasquini E, Doglietto F et al (2006) The endoscopic extended transsphenoidal approach for craniopharyngiomas. Neurosurgery 59:ONS75–ONS83; discussion ONS75-83

Gardner PA, Prevedello DM, Kassam AB et al (2008a) The evolution of the endonasal approach for craniopharyngiomas. J Neurosurg 108:1043–1047

Gardner PA, Kassam AB, Snyderman CH et al (2008b) Outcomes following endoscopic, expanded endonasal resection of suprasellar craniopharyngiomas: a case series. J Neurosurg 109:6–16

Giordano D (1897) Compendio di chirurgia operatoria. Unione Tipografico-Editrice Torinese, Torino, pp 101–104

Griffith HB, Veerapen R (1987) A direct transnasal approach to the sphenoid sinus. Technical note. J Neurosurg 66:140–142

Guiot G, Thibaut B, Bourreau M (1959) Extirpation of hypophyseal adenomas by trans-septal and trans-sphenoidal approaches. Ann Otolaryngol 76:1017–1031

Hadad G, Bassagasteguy L, Carrau RL et al (2006) A novel reconstructive technique after endoscopic expanded endonasal approaches: vascular pedicle nasoseptal flap. Laryngoscope 116:1882–1886

Hader WJ, Steinbok P, Hukin J, Fryer C (2000) Intratumoral therapy with bleomycin for cystic craniopharyngiomas in children. Pediatr Neurosurg 33:211–218

Halstead AE (1910) Remarks on the operative treatment of tumors of the hypophysis with the report of two cases operated on by an oro-nasal method. Surg Gynecol Obstet 10:494–502

Hamilton JK, Conwell LS, Syme C et al (2011) Hypothalamic obesity following craniopharyngioma surgery: results of a pilot trial of combined Diazoxide and metformin therapy. Int J Pediatr Endocrinol 2011:417949

Hasegawa T, Kondziolka D, Hadjipanayis CG et al (2004) Management of cystic craniopharyngiomas with phosphorus-32 intracavitary irradiation. Neurosurgery 54:813–820

Hochenegg J (1908) The operative cure of acromegaly by removal of hypophysial tumor. Ann Surg 48:781

Honegger J, Tatagiba M (2008) Craniopharyngioma surgery. Pituitary 11:361–373

Honegger J, Buchfelder M, Fahlbusch R (1999) Surgical treatment of craniopharyngiomas: endocrinological results. J Neurosurg 90:251–257

Horsley V (1906) On the technique of operations on the central nervous system. Br Med J 2:411–423

Huk WJ, Mahlstedt J (1983) Intracystic radiotherapy (90Y) of craniopharyngiomas: CT-guided stereotaxic implantation of indwelling drainage system. AJNR Am J Neuroradiol 4:803–806

Jane JA Jr, Kiehna E, Payne SC et al (2010a) Early outcomes of endoscopic transsphenoidal surgery for adult craniopharyngiomas. Neurosurg Focus 28:E9

Jane JA Jr, Prevedello DM, Alden TD et al (2010b) The transsphenoidal resection of pediatric craniopharyngiomas: a case series. J Neurosurg Pediatr 5:49–60

Jho HD, Carrau R (1997) Endoscopic endonasal transsphenoidal surgery: experience with 50 patients. J Neurosurg 87:44–51

Julow J, Backlund EO, Lanyi F et al (2007) Long-term results and late complications after intra-cavitary yttrium-90 colloid irradiation of recurrent cystic craniopharyngiomas. Neurosurgery 61:288–295

Kaptain GJ, Vincent DA, Sheehan JP et al (2001) Transsphenoidal approaches for the extracapsu-lar resection of midline suprasellar and anterior cranial base lesions. Neurosurgery 49:94–100; discussion 100–101

Karavitaki N, Brufani C, Warner JT et al (2005) Craniopharyngiomas in children and adults: sys-tematic analysis of 121 cases with long-term follow-up. Clin Endocrinol (Oxf) 62:397–409

Kassam AB, Thomas A, Carrau RL et al (2008) Endoscopic reconstruction of the cranial base using a pedicled nasoseptal flap. Neurosurgery 63:ONS44–ONS52

Kern EB, Pearson BW, McDonald TJ, Laws ER Jr (1979) The transseptal approach to lesions of the pituitary and parasellar regions. Laryngoscope 89:1–34

Kickingereder P, Maarouf M, El Majdoub F et al (2012) Intracavitary brachytherapy using stereotactically applied phosphorus-32 colloid for treatment of cystic craniopharyngiomas in 53 patients. J Neurooncol 109:365–374

Kim EH, Ahn JY, Kim SH (2011) Technique and outcome of endoscopy-assisted microscopic extended transsphenoidal surgery for suprasellar craniopharyngiomas. J Neurosurg 114:1338–1349

Komotar RJ, Roguski M, Bruce JN (2009) Surgical management of craniopharyngiomas. J Neurooncol 92:283–296

Komotar RJ, Starke RM, Raper DM et al (2012) Endoscopic endonasal compared with micro-scopic transsphenoidal and open transcranial resection of craniopharyngiomas. World Neurosurg 77:329–341

Laffond C, Dellatolas G, Alapetite C et al (2012) Quality-of-life, mood and executive functioning after childhood craniopharyngioma treated with surgery and proton beam therapy. Brain Inj 26:270–281

Laws ER Jr (1980) Transsphenoidal microsurgery in the management of craniopharyngioma. J Neurosurg 52:661–666

Laws ER (1987) Craniopharyngiomas in children and young adults. Prog Exp Tumor Res 30:335–340

Laws ER Jr (1994) Transsphenoidal removal of craniopharyngioma. Pediatr Neurosurg 21(Suppl 1):57–63

Laws ER Jr (1997) Craniopharyngioma: transsphenoidal surgery. Curr Ther Endocrinol Metab 6:35–38

Laws ER Jr, Jane JA Jr (2010) Craniopharyngioma. J Neurosurg Pediatr 5:27–28; discussion 28–29

Laws ER Jr, Morris AM, Maartens N (2003) Gliadel for pituitary adenomas and craniopharyngio-mas. Neurosurgery 53:255–269

Leksell LLK (1952) A Therapeutic trial with radioactive isotopes in cystic brain tumours. Radioisotope techniques. J Med Physiol Appl 4:1–4

Leng LZ, Greenfield JP, Souweidane MM et al (2012) Endoscopic, endonasal resection of cranio-pharyngiomas: analysis of outcome including extent of resection, cerebrospinal fluid leak, return to preoperative productivity, and body mass index. Neurosurgery 70:110–123

Liu W, Fang Y, Cai B et al (2012) Intracystic bleomycin for cystic craniopharyngiomas in children (abridged republication of cochrane systematic review). Neurosurgery 71:909–915

Maira G, Anile C, Rossi GF et al (1995) Surgical treatment of craniopharyngiomas: an evaluation of the transsphenoidal and pterional approaches. Neurosurgery 36:715–724

Maira G, Anile C, Albanese A et al (2004) The role of transsphenoidal surgery in the treatment of craniopharyngiomas. J Neurosurg 100:445–451

Matson DD, Crigler JF Jr (1969) Management of craniopharyngioma in childhood. J Neurosurg 30:377–390

Mottolese C, Stan H, Hermier M et al (2001) Intracystic chemotherapy with bleomycin in the treatment of craniopharyngiomas. Childs Nerv Syst 17:724–730

Müller HL, Gebhardt U, Wessel V, Schröder S et al (2007) First experiences with laparoscopic adjustable gastric banding (LAGB) in the treatment of patients with childhood craniopharyngioma and morbid obesity. Klin Padiatr 219:323–325

Oskouian RJ, Samii A, Laws ER Jr (2006) The craniopharyngioma. Front Horm Res 34:105–126

Page-Wilson G, Wardlaw SL, Khandji AG et al (2012) Hypothalamic obesity in patients with craniopharyngioma: treatment approaches and the emerging role of gastric bypass surgery. Pituitary 15:84–92

Prabhu VC, Brown HG (2005) The pathogenesis of craniopharyngiomas. Childs Nerv Syst 21:622–627

Samii M, Bini W (1991) Surgical treatment of craniopharyngiomas. Zentralbl Neurochir 52:17–23

Shapiro K, Till K, Grant DN (1979) Craniopharyngiomas in childhood. A rational approach to treatment. J Neurosurg 50:617–623

Spaziante R, De Divitiis E, Irace C et al (1989) Management of primary or recurring grossly cystic craniopharyngiomas by means of draining systems. Topic review and 6 case reports. Acta Neurochir 97:95–106

Szeifert GT, Julow J, Slowik F et al (1990) Pathological changes in cystic craniopharyngiomas following intracavital 90yttrium treatment. Acta Neurochir 102:14–18

Teo C (2005) Application of endoscopy to the surgical management of craniopharyngiomas. Childs Nerv Syst 21:696–700

Van den Berge JH, Blaauw G et al (1992) Intracavitary brachytherapy of cystic craniopharyngiomas. J Neurosurg 77:545–550

von Eiselsberg AvF-H L (1907) Uber die operative behandlung der tumoren der hypophysisgegend. Neurol Centralblatt 26:994–1001

Weiner HL, Wisoff JH, Rosenberg ME et al (1994) Craniopharyngiomas: a clinicopathological analysis of factors predictive of recurrence and functional outcome. Neurosurgery 35:1001–1010; discussion 1010–1001

Weiss MH (1987) Transnasal transsphenoidal approach. In: Apuzzo ML (ed) Surgery of the third ventricle. Williams and Wilkins, Baltimore, pp 476–494

Wilson WR, Khan A, Laws ER Jr (1990) Transseptal approaches for pituitary surgery. Laryngoscope 100:817–819

Yamada S, Fukuhara N, Oyama K et al (2010) Surgical outcome in 90 patients with craniopharyngioma: an evaluation of transsphenoidal surgery. World Neurosurg 74:320–330

Yasargil MG, Curcic M, Kis M et al (1990) Total removal of craniopharyngiomas. Approaches and long-term results in 144 patients. J Neurosurg 73:3–11

Young SC, Zimmerman RA, Nowell M et al (1987) Giant cystic craniopharyngiomas. Neuroradiology 29:468–473

Zada G, Cappabianca P (2010) Transsphenoidal surgery for craniopharyngiomas: the lessons of experience, timing, and restraint. World Neurosurg 74:256–258

Zada G, Lin N, Ojerholm E, Ramkissoon S et al (2010) Craniopharyngioma and other cystic epithelial lesions of the sellar region: a review of clinical, imaging, and histopathological relationships. Neurosurg Focus 28:E4

Zada G, Agarwalla PK, Mukundan S et al (2011) The neurosurgical anatomy of the sphenoid sinus and sellar floor in endoscopic transsphenoidal surgery. J Neurosurg 114:1319–1330

Zona G, Spaziante R (2006) Management of cystic craniopharyngiomas in childhood by a transsphenoidal approach. J Pediatr Endocrinol Metab 19(Suppl 1):381–388

Surgical Approach to Craniopharyngiomas: Transcranial Routes

5

Pietro Mortini, Filippo Gagliardi, Michele Bailo, and Marco Losa

Abstract

The optimal treatment of patients with craniopharyngioma remains controversial because an effective balanced protocol between aggressive therapy and reducing adverse sequelae is still lacking.

Radical resection is considered the therapy of choice for primary treatment, being associated with the best outcome in terms of survival and recurrence-free survival.

Transcranial surgery is performed in case of purely suprasellar or large intra-suprasellar dumbbell-shaped tumors, with extension toward the third ventricle and hypothalamus, subfrontal, retrochiasmatic, and retro-sellar regions.

Transcranial approaches comprise the frontopterional, the fronto-orbito-zygomatic (FOZ), and the combined interhemispheric subcommissural trans-laminaterminalis approach (CISTA).

The most relevant anatomic elements influencing the extent of resection and potential effectiveness of surgery, as well as the risk of surgical morbidity in craniopharyngioma surgery are tumor relationships with the third ventricle and hypothalamus, arachnoid plane and pia mater layer, optic pathways, pituitary stalk and vascular structures.

We discuss and comparatively analyze the role of FOZ, and CISTA in terms of indication, peculiar features and technique in the surgical treatment of craniopharyngiomas.

P. Mortini, MD • F. Gagliardi, MD (✉) • M. Bailo, MD • M. Losa, MD
Department of Neurosurgery and Gamma Knife Radiosurgery, Vita-Salute University, San Raffaele Scientific Institute, Milan, Italy
e-mail: gagliardi.filippo@hsr.it

© Springer International Publishing Switzerland 2016
A. Lania et al. (eds.), *Diagnosis and Management of Craniopharyngiomas: Key Current Topics*, DOI 10.1007/978-3-319-22297-4_5

5.1   Introduction

The best treatment option in patients harboring craniopharyngiomas (CFGs) still remains a matter of debate in the literature (Amacher 1980; Baskin and Wilson 1986; Bloom 1975; Carmel et al. 1982; Fischer et al. 1985; Hoff and Patterson 1972; Hoffman et al. 1977; Kahn et al. 1973; Katz 1975; Kramer 1976; Kramer et al. 1968, 1961; Lichter et al. 1977; Manaka et al. 1985; Matson 1964; Matson and Crigler 1969; McMurry et al. 1977; Michelsen et al. 1972; Muller and Morley 1976; Richmond et al. 1980; Sharma et al. 1974; Shillito 1976; Sweet 1976). The gold standard in the management of primary lesions is widely considered the radical surgical removal (Mortini et al. 2011; Sainte-Rose et al. 2005), which has been demonstrated to be associated with the best outcome in terms of overall and progression-free survival (Karavitaki et al. 2006; Mortini et al. 2011).

The extent of surgical resection mainly depends on tumor location and size, the calcification rate and the presence of hydrocephalus and neurovascular structures invasion. In large series, the rate of radical surgery widely ranges from 18 to 84 % of cases (Mortini et al. 2012).

On the other hand, extensive excision might be associated with notable perioperative morbidity and mortality, which is reported ranging from 1.7 to 5.4 % of cases (Mortini et al. 2012) and which is mainly due to tight adherences of the lesion toward the pituitary gland, hypothalamic axis and optic pathways, as well as to approach related intrinsic morbidity (Duff et al. 2000;   Karavitaki et al. 2005; Karavitaki et al. 2006; Kim et al. 2001).

Over the years many different microsurgical and endoscopic approaches have been developed for the resection of CFGs, which can be performed either as a single or in a combined staged procedure (Bartlett 1971; Baskin and Wilson 1986; Carpenter et al. 1937; Ciric and Cozzens 1980; Erdheim 1903; Fujitsu et al. 1994; Kanno et al. 1989; Laws 1980; Yasargil et al. 1990).

Among transcranial approaches, the orbito-zygomatic, (Fujitsu and Kuwabara 1986; Fujitsu et al. 1994; Gonzalez et al. 2002; Komotar et al. 2009; Lemole et al. 2003; Liu et al. 2005; Zabramski et al. 1998) the pterional, (Choux and Lena 1998; Fujitsu et al. 1994; Kanno et al. 1989; Komotar et al. 2009; Liu et al. 2005; Maira et al. 2000; Yasargil et al. 1990) the transpetrosal, (Al-Mefty et al. 2008; Fujitsu et al. 1994; Komotar et al. 2009) the transcortical-transventricular, (Choux and Lena 1998; Fujitsu et al. 1994; Kanno et al. 1989; Komotar et al. 2009; Liu et al. 2005; Tsutsumi et al. 1991) the transcallosal-transventricular (Komotar et al. 2009; Shucart 1987) and more recently the endoscopic approaches (Komotar et al. 2009; Schwartz et al. 2008) have been proposed for the resection of these tumors. Various combinations of the aforementioned approaches have been also described such as the subtemporal-transpetrosal, (Hakuba et al. 1985; Komotar et al. 2009) the pterional-transcallosal, (Komotar et al. 2009; Konovalov 1998; Liu et al. 2005) and the pterional-subfrontal (Komotar et al. 2009; Samii and Tatagiba 1997).

In our experience, according to previously published surgical results, in case of CFGs with large suprasellar extension, a combination of the trans-sylvian, subfrontal and interhemispheric translaminaterminalis corridors are needed to effective and safety approach the tumor (Mortini et al. 2011).

In the present chapter we discuss and comparatively analyze the role of FOZ and CISTA in terms of peculiar features and technique in the surgical treatment of large CFGs.

5.2   Anatomic Consideration for Surgical Planning

Surgical plan in tailoring the best treatment strategy to resect a CFG needs to take into consideration some critical aspects. Notably, the most relevant anatomic elements influencing the extent of resection and potential effectiveness of surgery, as well as the risk of surgical morbidity in CFG surgery, are tumor relationships with the third ventricle and hypothalamus, arachnoid plane and pia mater layer, optic pathways, pituitary stalk, and vascular structures (Mortini et al. 2012).

Particularly, the most important aspects to take into consideration by planning the surgery are tumor relationships toward walls and floor of the third ventricle. Understanding these relationships is indeed mandatory to perform a radical resection, minimizing the risk of damages to hypothalamic structures (Mortini et al. 2012). This aspect is still a matter of debate. Some authors indeed denied the existence of intraventricular craniopharyngiomas, defining them as pseudo-intraventricular craniopharyngiomas (Hoffman et al. 1992; Van Den Bergh and Brucher 1970). Contrarily, some others define intraventricular tumor as a distinct pathological entity (Sweet 1988).

CFGs can be also classified based on the relationships between the tumor, the arachnoid, and the pia mater planes (Ciric and Cozzens 1980). According to this classification system, tumors classified as intrapial-intraventricular are highly invasive and extremely difficult to remove. Besides, lesions with intrapial subarachnoidal extension are still invasive and usually firmly adherent to hypothalamic structures. Contrarily, the extrapial intra-arachnoidal CFGs can be, more frequently, radically removed. When the origin of the tumor is below the infundibular area, the lesion is usually bilobated; in this case CFG are classified as intra-arachnoidal in the supradiaphragmatic part and extra-arachnoidal into the sellar part. The last variant as described by Ciric and Cozzens are intrasellar CFGs, which are fully extra-arachnoidal, thus feasible for transsphenoidal resection (Ciric and Cozzens 1980).

Some other authors classified craniopharyngiomas according to the relationships of the tumor with the walls of the third ventricle. The first type is located both into the sellar and suprasellar region. A thick capsule, separated from the ventricular floor by an arachnoidal layer, forms the superior part of the lesion. This type of tumor can be radically removed without damaging the ventricular floor. The second type is purely supradiaphragmatic and can be extraventricular, intraventricular, or both. The suprasellar extraventricular CFGs can be extrapial and separated from the ventricular floor, being either pre-chiasmatic or retrochiasmatic. Suprasellar intraventricular lesions are usually tight adherent to mamillary bodies and infundibulum.

In this case radical resection can be challenging. Most of these tumors are retrochiasmatic (Mortini et al. 2012).

Other authors observed that CFGs use to be much more tightly adherent to the floor of the third ventricle in the area of the tuber cinereum, while elsewhere meningeal layers usually cover the tumor separating it from the hypothalamus. In these cases radical removal is often possible, without damages to the ventricular floor (Hoffman et al. 1992).

CFG relationships with the floor of the third ventricle might be different based on the consistence of the upper part of the lesion. Cystic tumors usually present a layer of connective tissue separating cyst's wall from the hypothalamus, which is not present in solid lesions. This finding explains the different surgical results obtained, according to tumor characteristics (Kobayashi et al. 2005; Sweet 1988).

Some authors described as particularly critical the presence of adherence to the anterior-inferior part of the hypothalamus, making the tumor in these cases impossible to be separated from nervous tissue (Yasargil et al. 1990).

In some other studies, it has been stated that tumors usually do not firmly adhere to the floor of the ventricle, which is at the end only invaginated by the lesion, and can be safety separated. On the other side, in case of tumors with intraventricular extension, ventricular walls are often deeply infiltrated and radical removal is often not feasible (Choux et al. 1991).

Tumor contacts with the optic pathways are further critical aspect in CFG surgery. Sometimes chiasm and optic nerves are compressed and dislocated; the vascular supply is intact and should be preserved during surgery. Nevertheless, in case of large tumors, it can be difficult to distinguish arterial feedings to the optic apparatus and those supplying the lesion (Mortini et al. 2011).

Many authors agree that the pituitary stalk is frequently invaded by the tumor and therefore should be divided in order to avoid potential recurrence (Mortini et al. 2011; Sweet 1988). However, in patients with normal preoperative pituitary function, if the lesion is separated from the stalk, it can be preserved, without increasing risk of recurrence (Mortini et al. 2012).

Nevertheless, the section of the pituitary stalk should not be considered as a major consequence of surgery. Nevertheless, it has to be emphasized that patients with adequate substitution therapies may have normal life expectancy (Mortini et al. 2011).

Finally, adherence between CFGs and major vessels is one of the main factors limiting the extent of resection. The carotid artery as well as its collateral branches might be encased or infiltrated by the tumor; however, arteries are usually separated from the lesion by an arachnoidal layer, making the dissection usually feasible (Choux et al. 1991).

5.3 Surgical Indications

The transcranial approaches are indicated in case of purely suprasellar or large intra-suprasellar dumbbell-shaped tumors, with extension toward the third ventricle and hypothalamus and the subfrontal, retrochiasmatic, retro-sellar regions (Alleyne et al. 2002; Goel et al. 2004; Mortini et al. 2007, 2013, 2005; Mortini and Giovanelli 2002).

In the first years of our surgical experience, the most used lateral transcranial approach was the frontopterional trans-sylvian route with its further translaminaterminalis extension. For deeply seated lesions growing into the third ventricle with large cranial extension, the interhemispheric anterior transcallosal route was preferred.

Since the late 1990s the fronto-orbito-zygomatic (FOZ) route (Ahmadi et al. 1985; Mortini and Giovanelli 2002; Mortini et al. 2007) together with its further development, the CISTA, (Mortini et al. 2013) progressively replaced the frontopterional and the transcallosal approaches. Cranial base techniques provide excellent surgical exposure of sellar and parasellar areas, with the possibility of optic nerve decompression, minimizing the need for brain retraction and neural tissue sacrifice (Alaywan and Sindou 1990; Fujitsu and Kuwabara 1985, 1986; Gonzalez et al. 2002; Mortini et al. 2007; Mortini and Giovanelli 2002).

5.4 Surgical Anatomy

In this section, we will focus the subject into the technical description of the FOZ approach with its further development, recently described by us as combined interhemispheric subcommissural translaminaterminalis approach (CISTA) (Mortini et al. 2013).

Surgical results are summarized in Table 5.1 (De Vile et al. 1996; Gonc et al. 2004; Kim et al. 2001; Lee et al. 2008; Merchant et al. 2002; Shi et al. 2008; Shirane et al. 2005; Stripp et al. 2004) and compared with the major series reported in the literature.

The FOZ approach and in its variant CISTA allow for an excellent visualization of the ipsilateral inter-optic, optic-carotid, and carotid-oculomotor windows, as well as the retro-carotid space, the posterior clinoid, the basilar apex, and the suprasellar region.

The visualization of the retrochiasmatic area provides a good control on the posterior circulation, enabling a safer dissection of tumor arterial feeders and perforating branches directed to the posterior optic pathways (Mortini et al. 2013).

The orbitotomy minimizes the need for brain retraction and widens the working and maneuverability areas (Gagliardi et al. 2014; Liu et al. 2005; Mortini et al. 2013; Mortini and Giovanelli 2002). Orbital roof removal provides direct access to the optic-chiasmatic cistern and to the suprasellar area through the unilateral subfrontal corridor and, after the opening of the Sylvian fissure, to the optic-carotid cistern (Lemole et al. 2003).

In the CISTA, the extension of the frontotemporal craniotomy up to the midline allows to use the basal unilateral interhemispheric subcallosal route to control the suprasellar component of the tumor (Fujitsu et al. 1994; Kanno et al. 1989; Oka et al. 1985; Shibuya et al. 1996; Tsutsumi et al. 1991; Yasui et al. 1992).

The opening of the lamina terminalis provides access to the third ventricle without any sacrifice of neural functional tissue (Shibuya et al. 1996; Suzuki et al. 1984). Subcommissural translaminaterminalis approach to the third ventricle minimizes

Table 5.1 Review of the literature

Study	No.	Mean age (year)	FU (year)	Children (%)	Tumor size (cm)	Preop hydrocephalus (%)	Preop visual deficit (%)	Postop CT/MRI	Radical Removal (%)	Surgical mortality (%)	Postop DI (%)
Hoffman et al. (1992)	50	9.4	4.9	100	N/A	48	58	CT/MRI	90	2	93
De Vile et al. (1996)	75	6.6	6.4	100	>3.5 (51 %)	54.1	N/A	CT/MRI	40	0	80
Kim et al. (2001)	36	7.3	4.3	100	>3 (100 %)	69.4	N/A	CT/MRI	100	0	94
Merchant et al. (2002)	30	8.6	6.1	100	>3.5 (51 %)	23	N/A	N/A	27	0	50
Stripp et al. (2004)	76	8.5	7.6	100	N/A	N/A	56.6	CT/MRI	62	1	80
Gonc et al. (2004)	66	4.2	5.1	100	N/A	46.2	N/A	CT/MRI	31	2	52
Shirane et al. (2005)	42	N/A	5	50	N/A	N/A	N/A	N/A	71	0	52
Lee et al. (2008)	66	8.0	7.2	100	N/A	N/A	N/A	CT/MRI	N/A	0	67
Shi et al. (2008)	309	9/36 (Ch/Ad)	2.1	16.2	3.5 (mean)	37.8	43	CT/MRI	89	3.9	53
Mean	83.3	7.5	5.4	85.1	N/A	46.4	52.5	N/A	63.8	1.0	69
Current series	102	35	6.3	27	3 (mean)	N/A	82.4	MRI	75.8	2.9	76

Study	Visual improvement (%)	Visual worsening (%)	Postop hypopituitarism (%)	Postop RT (%)	Overall survival (%)	Relapse (%)	Relapse after radical removal (%)	5-year PFS (%)	10-year PFS (%)
Hoffman et al. (1992)	36	41	N/A	0	98	34	29	N/A	N/A
De Vile et al. (1996)	N/A	N/A	99	51	80	41	10	N/A	N/A
Kim et al. (2001)	N/A	25	100	0	89	36	39	55	N/A
Merchant et al. (2002)	N/A	17	97	77	97	37	38	N/A	N/A
Stripp et al. (2004)	21	15	N/A	56	89	N/A	N/A	63	53
Gonc et al. (2004)	N/A	N/A	100	54.5	80	56	41	N/A	N/A
Shirane et al. (2005)	N/A	N/A	81	N/A	93	38	20	N/A	N/A
Lee et al. (2008)	N/A	N/A	N/A	N/A	97	N/A	N/A	N/A	N/A
Shi et al. (2008)	42	5.5	N/A	N/A	94	14/75	14	75	N/A
Mean	33.0	20.7	95.4	39.8	90.8	40.3	27.3	64.3	53.0
Current series	63.7	17.7	96	9.6	92.2	23.4	15.5	76.6	64.6

A adults, *Ch* children, *DI* diabetes insipidus, *FU* follow-up, *preop* preoperative, *PFS* progression-free survival, *postop* postoperative, *RT* radiotherapy the risk of damage to the frontal lobes, corpus callosum, and fornix as compared to traditional interhemispheric transcallosal approaches to the same area (Fujitsu et al. 1994; Suzuki et al. 1984).

Some authors suggested the division of the ACoA, during the interhemispheric translaminaterminalis approach (Asano 1989; Fujitsu et al. 1994; Shibuya et al. 1996; Suzuki et al. 1984).

According to our experience, ACoA division is unnecessary. To widen the surgical field, we described two alternative ways of opening the lamina terminalis, which can also be combined. The first route is obtained passing on the midline below and above the ACoA, between the two A1 and the two A2 segments, respectively. The second route is carried on the vascular angle defined by the lateral surface of A1 and A2 artery segments, which is free from major perforating branches and can be easily widen by retracting the vessels (Mortini et al. 2013). This route can be performed safely in any cases of the described arterial configurations (Yasargil 1984).

5.5 Technique

5.5.1 FOZ

The patient is positioned supine with the head fixed in a Mayfield head holder. The neck is slightly extended (10°) and elevated. The head is rotated at the contralateral side of about 30°. The maxillary eminence is the highest point in the surgical field.

Skin incision, running from ear to ear far behind the hairline, is performed and the skin flap together with pericranium is reflected anteriorly, taking care to preserve the supraorbital nerve and artery.

The interfascial dissection of the temporalis muscle is carried out and it is elevated through subperiosteal dissection as a separate layer and reflected anteriorly and inferiorly (Yasargil et al. 1987).

A frontotemporal craniotomy is performed with a frontal extension as low as possible on the orbital rim, just lateral to the supraorbital notch. The bone flap is elevated identifying the superior orbital fissure just medial to the orbito-meningeal artery.

The orbitotomy is performed making first a sagittal cut on the superior orbital rim close to the supraorbital foramen and an axial one on the lateral orbital rim, just superior to the body of the zygoma, directed toward the inferior orbital fissure. The osteotomies are then connected using a high-speed drill, obtaining a free orbito-zygomatic bone flap. In case of frontal sinus opening, a pedicled galeal flap should be harvest and reflected to close it.

At this point of the procedure, the extradural optic nerve decompression can be performed by unroofing the optic canal with a high-speed drill and exposing the optic dural sheet.

The dura is tented to the margins of the bone flap with 3.0 silk sutures, and it is opened in a curvilinear C-shape fashion across the Sylvian fissure with its base along the periorbita.

The dural flap is reflected over the orbital fat and gently put in tension by dural stitches in order to displace the orbital contents downward to obtain an unobstructed view of the optic nerve without any brain retraction.

The trans-sylvian corridor is used opening the sylvian fissure and it is enlarged toward the lateral aspect of the subfrontal corridor, exposing the ipsilateral optic-carotid, and the carotid-oculomotor windows, as well as the inter-optic and retro-carotid space, the posterior clinoid region, the basilar apex, and the suprasellar region (Fujitsu and Kuwabara 1985, 1986; Fujitsu et al. 1994; Gonzalez et al. 2002; Komotar et al. 2009; Lemole et al. 2003; Liu et al. 2005; Zabramski et al. 1998).

5.5.2 CISTA

The frontotemporal craniotomy usually done in case of FOZ approach is enlarged till the midline to expose the superior sagittal sinus.

After the craniotomy, an appropriate orbital osteotomy is carried out and the optic canal is unroofed to obtain extradural optic nerve decompression.

The dura is widely opened in a curvilinear C-shape fashion across the Sylvian fissure, toward the midline. The dural flap is downward reflected and put in tension to depress the orbital contents.

The frontal lobe is gently separated from the falx and the contralateral cortex, opening the interhemispheric fissure toward the lamina terminalis.

The A1 and A2 segments, the ACoA, and the posterior edge of the optic chiasm are exposed. The lamina terminalis can be sequentially opened on the midline below the ACoA between the two A1 segments and above the ACoA between the two A2 segments. Another route distal to the ACoA corresponds to the vascular angle formed by the lateral surfaces of A1 and the A2 segments. Suprasellar area is controlled assessing the whole cavity of the third ventricle.

5.6 Clinical Series

5.6.1 Patient Population

Between 1990 and 2014, at our Institution, 102 patients underwent transcranial surgery for craniopharyngioma. Mean age at surgery was 35.0 ± 1.8 years, ranging between 6 and 69 years.

Childhood cases, defined as an age <18 years, represented 27.5 % of all cases (28 of 102 patients).

Histological analysis of tumor specimens confirmed the presence of craniopharyngioma in all cases. Based on morphological appearance, 92 tumors (90.2 %) were classified as adamantinomatous subtype and 10 tumors (9.8 %) as papillary subtype.

Invasion of the tumor into the surrounding nervous tissue occurred in 31 patients (30.4 %).

5.6.2 Early Postoperative Results

Visual function was impaired before surgery in 84 patients of the 102 (82.4 %). Forty-five out of these 82 patients (53.6 %) had a visual field defect only, while the remaining 39 patients (46.4 %) also had an impaired visual acuity. Ninety-six patients had postoperative information available.

Visual function improved after surgery in 51 of 80 (63.7 %) with preoperative deficit and available postoperative information, remained unchanged in 16 patients (20.0 %), while worsened in some way in the remaining 13 patients (16.3 %). No postoperative blindness was recorded in any eye. Among the 16 patients with preoperative normal visual examination and available postoperative information, 12 patients (75.0 %) retained a normal function, while the remaining four patients (25.0 %) developed a permanent partial visual field defect.

Changes of endocrine function after surgery are reported for each single pituitary axis. Only patients with the available relevant information both before and after surgery were included in this analysis. At baseline, normal gonadal, thyroid, adrenal, or somatotroph function was present in 16 (21.9 %), 53 (54.1 %), 52 (53.1 %), and 18 (18.8 %) patients, respectively. A new defect of the corresponding pituitary axis occurred postoperatively in 11 (68.8 %), 45 (84.9 %), 44 (84.6 %), and 12 (66.7 %) of the patients, respectively. On the contrary, 57, 45, 46, and 24 patients had a preoperative deficit of gonadal, thyroid, adrenal, or somatotroph function, respectively, that did not recover after surgery. Sixty-seven patients had normal urinary concentrating ability before surgery and six of them (9.0 %) retained a normal function while the remaining 61 (91.0 %) had postoperative onset of diabetes insipidus. Of the 33 patients with preoperative diabetes insipidus, two patients (6.1 %) regained a normal urinary concentrating ability.

The first postoperative MRI showed residual tumor in 24 of the 99 patients who could be evaluated (24.2 %), whereas no tumor was demonstrable in the remaining 75 patients (75.8 %).

5.6.3 Tumor Recurrence

In the group of 24 patients with visible residual tumor, radiation therapy was performed in 9 cases (37.5 %). No patient without visible tumor remnant on postoperative MRI underwent radiotherapy. Therefore 9 out of 94 patients (9.6 %) underwent radiotherapy after surgical removal of the craniopharyngioma.

Analyses on tumor recurrence are restricted only to the 94 patients (92.2 %) in whom ≥ 2 neuroimaging studies are available during follow-up. The median follow-up for the 94 patients on active follow-up was 75 months (interquartile range, 37.5–142.5 months), and the median neuroradiological follow-up was 66.5 months (interquartile range, 35–137.5 months).

Recurrence of craniopharyngioma occurred in 22 of the 94 patients (23.4 %). Figure 5.1 shows that the risk of recurrence is higher in the first 5 years after surgery and then shows a plateau. The recurrence-free survival at 5 and 10 years was 76.6 % (95 % CI 66.8–85.4 %; Fig. 5.1) and 64.6 % (95 % CI 50.4–78.8 %), respectively. The presence of residual tumor after surgery was the strongest predictor of late

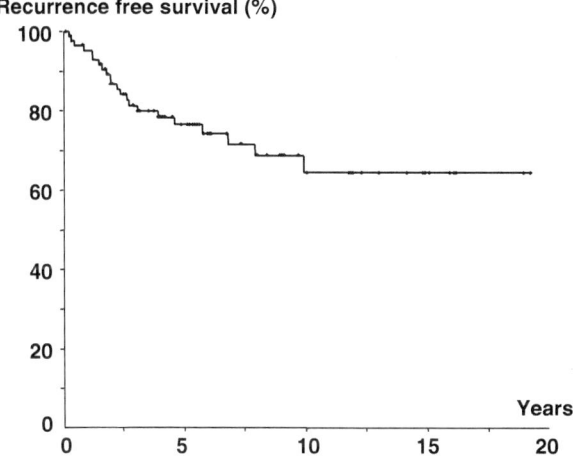

Fig. 5.1 Kaplan-Meier curve showing recurrence-free survival in the entire population

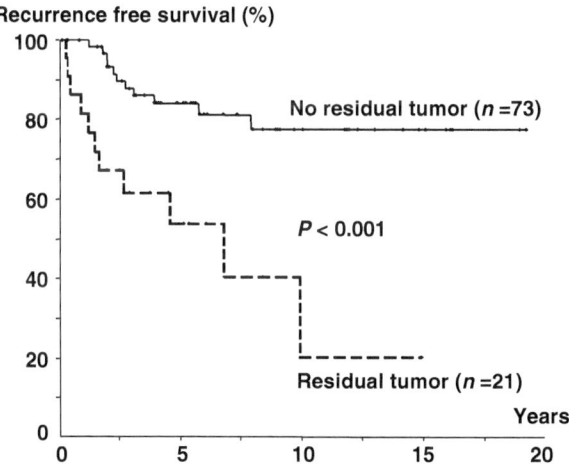

Fig. 5.2 Kaplan-Meier curve showing recurrence-free survival in patients with or without tumor recurrence

recurrence of the tumor (Fig. 5.2). The 5-year recurrence-free survival in patients with no residual tumor was 84.1 % (95 % CI 74.3–93.9 %) as compared with 53.8 % (95 % CI 31.1–76.5 %; $p < 0.001$; Fig. 5.2) in patients with residual tumor.

5.6.4   Further Treatments and Disease Status at Last Follow-Up

At the end of the follow-up period, control of tumor growth was obtained in all patients and there was no death attributable to progressive disease.

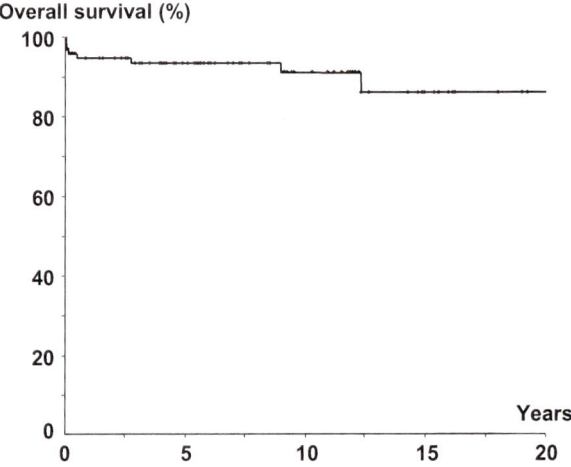

Fig. 5.3 Kaplan-Meier curve showing overall survival in the entire population

In the whole group of patients, there were five additional deaths at 2, 6, 33, 108, and 148 months after surgery. The cause of death was pulmonary embolism in one case, car accident in one case, and sepsis in one case and was unknown in two cases.

Figure 5.3 shows the overall survival of the 94 patients included into the study. The 5-year survival was 93.6 % (95 % CI 88.5–98.7 %) and the 10-year survival was 91.1 % (95 % CI 84.2–98.0 %).

References

Ahmadi J, North CM, Segall HD, Zee C-S, Weiss MH (1985) Cavernous sinus invasion by pituitary adenomas. AJNR 6:893–898

Al-Mefty O, Ayoubi S, Kadri PA (2008) The petrosal approach for the resection of retrochiasmatic craniopharyngiomas. Neurosurgery 62:ONS331–ONS335; discussion ONS335–336

Alaywan M, Sindou M (1990) Fronto-temporal approach with orbito-zygomatic removal surgical anatomy. Acta Neurochir (Wien) 104:79–83

Alleyne CH Jr, Barrow DL, Oyesiku NM (2002) Combined transsphenoidal and pterional craniotomy approach to giant pituitary tumors. Surg Neurol 57:380–390

Amacher AL (1980) Craniopharyngioma: the controversy regarding radiotherapy. Childs Brain 6:57–64

Asano T (1989) Interhemispheric, trans-lamina terminalis approach for craniopharyngioma. No Shinkei Geka 17:799

Bartlett JR (1971) Craniopharyngiomas--a summary of 85 cases. J Neurol Neurosurg Psychiatry 34:37–41

Baskin DS, Wilson CB (1986) Surgical management of craniopharyngiomas. A review of 74 cases. J Neurosurg 65:22–27

Bloom HJ (1975) Combined modality therapy for intracranial tumors. Cancer 35:111–120

Carmel PW, Antunes JL, Chang CH (1982) Craniopharyngiomas in children. Neurosurgery 11:382–389

Carpenter RC, Chamberlin GW, Frazier C (1937) The treatment of hypophyseal stalk tumors by evacuation and irradiation. Am J Roentgenol 38:162–177

Choux M, Lena G (1998) Craniopharyngioma. In: Apuzzo MLJ (ed) Surgery of the third ventricle, vol 2. Williams and Wilkins, Baltimore, pp 1143–1181

Choux M, Lena G, Genitori L (1991) [Craniopharyngioma in children]. Sociètè de neurochirurgie de lenguage franciase. 41° Congrès annuel, Lisbonne

Ciric IS, Cozzens JW (1980) Craniopharyngiomas: transsphenoidal method of approach--for the virtuoso only? Clin Neurosurg 27:169–187

De Vile CJ, Grant DB, Kendall BE et al (1996) Management of childhood craniopharyngioma: can the morbidity of radical surgery be predicted? J Neurosurg 85:73–81

Duff J, Meyer FB, Ilstrup DM et al (2000) Long-term outcomes for surgically resected craniopharyngiomas. Neurosurgery 46:291–302; discussion 302–395

Erdheim J (1903) Zur normalen und pathologischen Histologie der Glandula thyreoidea, parathyreoidea und Hypophysis. Beitr Pathol Anat Allge 33:158–236

Fischer EG, Welch K, Belli JA et al (1985) Treatment of craniopharyngiomas in children: 1972–1981. J Neurosurg 62:496–501

Fujitsu K, Kuwabara T (1985) Zygomatic approach for lesions in the interpeduncular cistern. J Neurosurg 62:340–343

Fujitsu K, Kuwabara T (1986) Orbitocraniobasal approach for anterior communicating artery aneurysms. Neurosurgery 18:367–369

Fujitsu K, Sekino T, Sakata K et al (1994) Basal interfalcine approach through a frontal sinusotomy with vein and nerve preservation: Technical note. J Neurosurg 80:575–579

Gagliardi F, Boari N, Roberti F et al (2014) Operability score: an innovative tool for quantitative assessment of operability in comparative studies on surgical anatomy. J Craniomaxillofac Surg 42(6):1000–4

Goel A, Nadkarni T, Muzumdar D et al (2004) Giant pituitary tumors: a study based on surgical treatment of 118 cases. Surg Neurol 61:436–445

Gonc EN, Yordam N, Ozon A, Alikasifoglu A, Kandemir N (2004) Endocrinological outcome of different treatment options in children with craniopharyngioma: a retrospective analysis of 66 cases. Pediatr Neurosurg 40:112–119

Gonzalez LF, Crawford NR, Horgan MA et al (2002) Working area and angle of attack in three cranial base approaches: pterional, orbitozygomatic, and maxillary extension of the orbitozygomatic approach. Neurosurgery 50:550–557

Hakuba A, Nishimura S, Inoue Y (1985) Transpetrosal-transtentorial approach and its application in the therapy of retrochiasmatic craniopharyngiomas. Surg Neurol 24:405–415

Hoff JT, Patterson RH Jr (1972) Craniopharyngiomas in children and adults. J Neurosurg 36:299–302

Hoffman HJ, De Silva M, Humphreys RP et al (1992) Aggressive surgical management of craniopharyngiomas in children. J Neurosurg 76:47–52

Hoffman HJ, Hendrick EB, Humphreys RP et al (1977) Management of craniopharyngioma in children. J Neurosurg 47:218–227

Kahn EA, Gosch HH, Seeger JF et al (1973) Forty-five years experience with the craniopharyngiomas. Surg Neurol 1:5–12

Kanno T, Kasama A, Shoda M et al (1989) A pitfall in the interhemispheric translamina terminalis approach for the removal of a craniopharyngioma. Significance of preserving draining veins. Part I. Clinical study. Surg Neurol 32:111–115

Karavitaki N, Brufani C, Warner JT et al (2005) Craniopharyngiomas in children and adults: systematic analysis of 121 cases with long-term follow-up. Clin Endocrinol (Oxf) 62: 397–409

Karavitaki N, Cudlip S, Adams CB et al (2006) Craniopharyngiomas. Endocr Rev 27:371–397

Katz EL (1975) Late results of radical excision of craniopharyngiomas in children. J Neurosurg 42:86–93

Kim SK, Wang KC, Shin SH et al (2001) Radical excision of pediatric craniopharyngioma: recurrence pattern and prognostic factors. Childs Nerv Syst 17:531–536; discussion 537

Kobayashi T, Kida Y, Mori Y, Hasegawa T (2005) Long-term results of gamma knife surgery for the treatment of craniopharyngioma in 98 consecutive cases. J Neurosurg 103:482–488

Komotar RJ, Roguski M, Bruce JN (2009) Surgical management of craniopharyngiomas. J Neurooncol 92:283–296

Konovalov AN (1998) Technique and strategies of direct surgical management of craniopharyngiomas. In: Apuzzo MLJ (ed) Surgery of the third ventricle, vol 2. Williams and Wilkins, Baltimore, pp 1133–1142

Kramer S (1976) Craniopharyngioma: the best treatment is conservative surgery and postoperative radiation therapy. In: Morley TP (ed) Current controversies in neurosurgery. WB Saunders, Philadelphia, pp 336–343

Kramer S, McKissock W, Concannon JP (1961) Craniopharyngiomas. Treatment by combined surgery and radiation therapy. J Neurosurg 18:217–226

Kramer S, Southard M, Mansfield CM (1968) Radiotherapy in the management of craniopharyngiomas: further experiences and late results. Am J Roentgenol Radium Ther Nucl Med 103:44–52

Laws ER Jr (1980) Transsphenoidal microsurgery in the management of craniopharyngioma. J Neurosurg 52:661–666

Lee YY, Wong TT, Fang YT et al (2008) Comparison of hypothalamopituitary axis dysfunction of intrasellar and third ventricular craniopharyngiomas in children. Brain Dev 30:189–194

Lemole GM Jr, Henn JS et al (2003) Modifications to the orbitozygomatic approach: technical note. J Neurosurg 99:924–930

Lichter AS, Wara WM, Sheline GE et al (1977) The treatment of craniopharyngiomas. Int J Radiat Oncol Biol Phys 2:675–683

Liu JK, Cole CD, Kestle JR et al (2005) Cranial base strategies for resection of craniopharyngioma in children. Neurosurg Focus 18:1–9

Maira G, Anile C, Colosimo C, Cabezas D (2000) Craniopharyngiomas of the third ventricle: trans-lamina terminalis approach. Neurosurgery 47:857–863; discussion 863–865

Manaka S, Teramoto A, Takakura K (1985) The efficacy of radiotherapy for craniopharyngioma. J Neurosurg 62:648–656

Matson DD (1964) Craniopharyngioma. Clin Neurosurg 10:116–129

Matson DD, Crigler JF Jr (1969) Management of craniopharyngioma in childhood. J Neurosurg 30:377–390

McMurry FG, Hardy RW Jr, Dohn DF et al (1977) Long term results in the management of craniopharyngiomas. Neurosurgery 1:238–241

Merchant TE, Kiehna EN, Sanford RA et al (2002) Craniopharyngioma: the St. Jude Children's Research Hospital experience 1984-2001. Int J Radiat Oncol Biol Phys 53:533–542

Michelsen WJ, Mount LA, Renaudin J (1972) Craniopharyngioma. A thirty-nine year survey. Acta Neurol Latinoam 18:100–106

Mortini P, Barzaghi R, Losa M et al (2007) Surgical treatment of giant pituitary adenomas: strategies and results in a series of 95 consecutive patients. Neurosurgery 60:993–1002; discussion 1003–1004

Mortini P, Gagliardi F, Boari N et al (2013) The combined interhemispheric subcommissural translaminaterminalis approach for large craniopharyngiomas. World Neurosurg 80:160–166

Mortini P, Giovanelli M (2002) Transcranial approaches to pituitary tumors. Oper Tech Neurosurg 5:239–251

Mortini P, Losa M, Barzaghi R et al (2005) Results of transsphenoidal surgery in a large series of patients with pituitary adenoma. Neurosurgery 56:1222–1233

Mortini P, Losa M, Gagliardi F (2012) Radical removal of Craniopharyngiomas. In: Hayat MA (ed) Tumors of the central nervous system. vol 9: lymphoma, supratentorial tumors, glioneuronal tumors, gangliogliomas, neuroblastoma in adults, astrocytomas, ependymomas, hemangiomas, and craniopharyngiomas. Springer Science & Business Media, Dordrecht

Mortini P, Losa M, Pozzobon G et al (2011) Neurosurgical treatment of craniopharyngioma in adults and children: early and long-term results in a large case series. J Neurosurg 114:1350–1359

Muller PJR, Morley TP (1976) Craniopharyngioma: results of surgical treatment without radiotherapy. In: Morley TP (ed) Current controversies in neurosurgery. WB Saunders, Philadelphia, pp 344–350

Oka K, Rhoton AL Jr, Barry M, Rodriguez R (1985) Microsurgical anatomy of the superficial veins of the cerebrum. Neurosurgery 17:711–748

Richmond IL, Wara WM, Wilson CB (1980) Role of radiation therapy in the management of craniopharyngiomas in children. Neurosurgery 6:513–517

Sainte-Rose C, Puget S, Wray A et al (2005) Craniopharyngioma: the pendulum of surgical management. Childs Nerv Syst 21:691–695

Samii M, Tatagiba M (1997) Surgical management of craniopharyngiomas: a review. Neurol Med Chir 37:141–149

Schwartz TH, Fraser JF, Brown S et al (2008) Endoscopic cranial base surgery: classification of operative approaches. Neurosurgery 62:991–1002; discussion 1002–1005

Sharma U, Tandon PN, Saxena KK et al (1974) Craniopharyngiomas treated by a combination of surgery and radiotherapy. Clin Radiol 25:13–17

Shi XE, Wu B, Fan T et al (2008) Craniopharyngioma: surgical experience of 309 cases in China. Clin Neurol Neurosurg 110:151–159

Shibuya M, Takayasu M, Suzuki Y et al (1996) Bifrontal basal interhemispheric approach to craniopharyngioma resection with or without division of the anterior communicating artery. J Neurosurg 84:951–956

Shillito JJ (1976) The treatment of craniopharyngiomas of childhood. In: Morley TP (ed) Current controversies in neurosurgery. WB Saunders, Philadelphia, pp 332–335

Shirane R, Hayashi T, Tominaga T (2005) Fronto-basal interhemispheric approach for craniopharyngiomas extending outside the suprasellar cistern. Childs Nerv Syst 21:669–678

Shucart W (1987) Anterior transcallosal and transcortical approaches. In: Apuzzo MLJ (ed) Surgery of the third ventricle. Williams and Wilkins, Baltimore, pp 303–325

Stripp DC, Maity A, Janss AJ et al (2004) Surgery with or without radiation therapy in the management of craniopharyngiomas in children and young adults. Int J Radiat Oncol Biol Phys 58:714–720

Suzuki J, Katakura R, Mori T (1984) Interhemispheric approach through the lamina terminalis to tumors of the anterior part of the third ventricle. Surg Neurol 22:157–163

Sweet WH (1976) Radical surgical treatment of craniopharyngioma. Clin Neurosurg 23:52–79

Sweet WH (1988) Craniopharyngiomas (with a note on Rathke's cleft or epithelial cyst and on suprasellar cyst). In: Schmidek H, Sweet WH (eds) Operative neurosurgical techniques: indications, methods, and results. Grune and Stratton, Orlando, pp 349–379

Tsutsumi K, Shiokawa Y, Sakai T et al (1991) Venous infarction following the interhemispheric approach in patients with acute subarachnoid hemorrhage. J Neurosurg 74:715–729

Van Den Bergh R, Brucher JM (1970) The transventricular approach in cranio-pharyngioma of the 3d ventricle. Neurosurgical and neuropathologic aspects. Neurochirurgie 16:51–65

Yasargil M (1984) Microneurosurgery, vol 1. Georg Thieme Verlag, Stuttgart

Yasargil MG, Curcic M, Kis M et al (1990) Total removal of craniopharyngiomas. Approaches and long-term results in 144 patients. J Neurosurg 73:3–11

Yasargil MG, Reichman MV, Kubik S (1987) Preservation of the frontotemporal branch of the facial nerve using the interfascial temporalis flap for pterional craniotomy: technical article. J Neurosurg 67:463–466

Yasui N, Nathal E, Fujiwara H, Suzuki A (1992) The basal interhemispheric approach for acute anterior communicating aneurysms. Acta Neurochir (Wien) 118:91–97

Zabramski JM, Kiris T, Sankhla SK et al (1998) Orbitozygomatic craniotomy: technical note. J Neurosurg 89:336–341

Radiotherapy and Radiosurgery for Craniopharyngiomas

6

Luca Attuati and Piero Picozzi

Abstract

At present, no firm consensus opinion exists concerning the appropriate management of craniopharyngioma, and no guidelines have been proposed, but radical resection is considered the primary choice for therapy. However, the majority of authors stated that successful management is determined by the ability to preserve independent social life and increasing survival while limiting symptomatic recurrence. In this view, the near-total resection followed by radiotherapy or radiosurgery on tumor remnant may be a suitable alternative to gross-total resection, with the aim of achieving tumor control without the endocrinological and behavioral morbidity associated with aggressive surgery.

6.1 Introduction

The term "craniopharyngioma" was first introduced by Harvey Cushing in 1932 (Cushing 1932) who described it as "one of the most baffling problems which confront the neurosurgeon."

Estimated occurrence is 0.13 % new cases per 100,000 persons/years (Ulfarsson et al. 2002). They account for 1–5 % (Mortini et al. 2011) of all primary

L. Attuati, MD • P. Picozzi, MD (✉)
Department of Neurosurgery, Gamma Knife Unit,
Humanitas Research Hospital, Rozzano, Italy
e-mail: piero.picozzi@humanitas.it

© Springer International Publishing Switzerland 2016   101
A. Lania et al. (eds.), *Diagnosis and Management of Craniopharyngiomas:
Key Current Topics*, DOI 10.1007/978-3-319-22297-4_6

intracranial tumors and 13 % (Samii and Tatagiba 1997; Rickert and Paulus 2001) in children. Distribution by age is bimodal, with peak incidence in children aged 5–14 years and adults aged 65–74 years; no definite genetic relationship has been found. Limiting the analysis only to adult patients, 16 years older and more, a study shows always a bimodal distribution, with two peaks ranging at about 16–22 and 35–52 (Lopez-Serna and Gomez-Amadorv 2012). No gender variance has been found, also if a slight male incidence (55 %) exists in all age groups. No genetic cause has been found, and very few familial cases have been reported (Karavitaki et al. 2006).

Craniopharyngiomas most frequently arise in the pituitary stalk and project into the hypothalamus. They are considered histologically benign, classified as WHO Grade I tumors, but local aggressivity and close proximity to delicate neural structures such as the hypothalamic–pituitary axis, thalamus and optic pathways make them one of the most challenging problems in current cranial surgery. This complex anatomical situation and the close relationship of radiation sensitive structures are also challenging for ancillary treatment such as radiotherapy or radiosurgery.

The first option in craniopharyngioma treatment is the surgical excision. There are two basic treatment lines proposed in literature: an aggressive approach and a more conservative one. The aggressive approach attempts gross-total resection at the diagnosis stage, while the second one combines a planned limited surgery followed by external beam irradiation.

Craniopharyngiomas often demonstrate an aggressive local behavior after surgery and may require adjuvant radiotherapy. Given the high rate of tumor recurrence also following gross-total resection, preventive postoperative radiotherapy has been proposed. A 3-year follow-up multivariate analysis in a German multicenter trial (Müller et al. 2010) has reported that irradiated patients had a lower risk of recurrence/progression compared with patients without irradiation and that waiting for recurrence carries a higher mortality rate.

Actually, no firm consensus opinion exists concerning the appropriate management of craniopharyngioma, and no guidelines have been proposed, but radical resection is considered the primary choice for therapy. However, the majority of authors stated that successful management is determined by the ability to preserve independent social life and increasing survival while limiting symptomatic recurrence.

In this view, the near-total resection followed by radiotherapy or radiosurgery on tumor remnant may be a suitable alternative to gross-total resection, with the aim of achieving tumor control without the endocrinologic and behavioral morbidity associated with aggressive surgery. However, radiotherapy is often not an option in case of very young children because of high rate of adverse effects due to damage to delicate neural structures playing a crucial role in thriving.

Malignant transformation into squamous cell carcinoma following irradiation has been documented both in adults and in children but is a rare event (Rodriguez et al. 2007).

External beam radiation may be utilized after partial resection surgery. Doses commonly utilized are in the range of 4500–5500 cGy delivered at 180 cGy/fraction. When applicable, radiosurgery on remnant tumor is reported to cause less local damages to surrounding structures while achieving a good tumor control.

Recurrence rates after gross-total resection were reported as 0–50 % (Liubinas et al. 2011; Clark et al. 2013). The most consistent reported feature predictive for recurrence of craniopharyngioma is the extent of resection at initial surgery. Statistical analysis demonstrates that the presence of residual tumor after surgery is the most probable cause of recurrence, while the age at the diagnosis does not seem to affect the occurrence rate, with the exception of very young patients with age less than 5 years. Other factors reported as being predictive for tumor recurrence include many causes, as tumor diameter, extrasellar extension, extension into the third ventricle, hydrocephalus, and tumors with high calcification rate (Liubinas et al. 2011).

It is mandatory to perform a postoperative MRI to evaluate the extent of resection and the presence of tumor remnant in order to plan postoperative radiotherapy or radiosurgery. Brain MRI scan should be planned 1–2 weeks following surgery for all patients, and patients with subtotal resections and candidates for external beam radiation therapy should start radiation within 3 weeks of surgery.

Neuroradiological follow-up as well as neurophtalmological and endocrinological evaluation should be performed every 3 months for the first postsurgical year, every 6 months for the second and third years, and yearly thereafter. Neurocognitive testing has to be considered for preoperative and postoperative patients as well as patients who have undergone subtotal resection followed by radiation (Di Pinto et al. 2010).

The management of recurrent craniopharyngioma remains one of the most difficult and controversial topics in neurosurgery, and the therapeutic decisions require a multidisciplinary approach (neurosurgeon, endocrinologist, neuro-ophthalmologist, and radiotherapist). In addition, the patient and their family must be involved explaining risks, limitations, and implications of the proposed treatment options.

Treatment options of recurrent craniopharyngioma include second surgery; intracystic bleomycin chemotherapy, if a cystic component is present; radiotherapy; and radiosurgery. Up to date, there is no proven role for chemotherapy in the treatment of craniopharyngioma and it remains experimental (Hargrave 2006).

Only with MRI follow-up recurrence can be accurately assessed. The advances in MRI techniques have improved the follow-up of craniopharyngioma, that is now more accurate and can demonstrate recurrence before clinical symptoms become evident, and a second treatment can be planned earlier. The radiological features of recurrent craniopharyngioma are similar to that of primary disease and differ for solid portion and cystic. For adamantinomatous craniopharyngiomas, the first portion is isointense to hyperintense on T1-weighted MRI, and the cystic area are hyperintense. In papillary craniopharyngiomas, there is a more uniform MRI appearance, hypointense on T1-weighted MRI with contrast enhancement of the cyst wall, and hyperintense on T2-weighted imaging.

6.2 Radiotherapy and Radiosurgery

The most disabling toxicity associated with aggressive primary surgery is hypothalamic damage leading to morbid obesity, sleep and temperature dysregulation, electrolyte disturbances, cognitive and behavioral abnormalities, and failure to thrive in children.

Given that radiotherapy is not associated with this risk because it preserves the structural integrity of the hypothalamus, it has become the preferred therapeutic option especially in case of tumor recurrence or substantial residual tumor.

Several radiotherapeutic modalities have been used in the past decades including conventional external beam radiation therapy, intensity-modulated radiation therapy, fractionated stereotactic RT, and proton beam RT, achieving a reasonable rates of tumor control. Doses commonly utilized are in the range of 4500–5500 cGy delivered at 180 cGy/fraction.

Iannalfi et al. (2013) has described and reviewed the role and results of radiotherapy on the treatment of craniopharyngiomas, presenting a complete review of published articles conducted using MEDLINE, Current Contents, and PubMed databases with different combination of terms.

Due to several factors (low incidence of tumor, lack of multidisciplinary team), literature data do not show homogeneity, especially data with large range of patient age. An early study by De Vile et al. (Di Pinto et al. 2010) showed a positive prognostic factor, and the already cited German study (Müller et al. 2010) reported a lower risk of recurrence, in patients submitted to RT after surgery.

Literature review demonstrates that survival rates after radiotherapy, both postoperative and primary alone, seem similar to those obtained by radical surgery, especially when analyzing groups with both gross and subtotal resections. The results are valid also considering clinical outcomes. Moreover, data do not suggest that patient age should influence the decision whether or not to use radiotherapy, excluding infants.

Trying to select the optimal dose delivered with conventional fractionation (i.e., 1.8–2 Gy/fraction), a difficulty arises from publications because radiotherapy techniques used are frequently not reported. Based on the publication data, Iannalfi et al. (2013) assumed that a proportion of patients were treated with two-dimensional radiotherapy and simple three-dimensional conformal techniques. Improvements in the accuracy of radiation delivery, due also to the introduction of stereotactic systems and image-guided radiotherapy, result in a reduction in the margin applied of the planned target volume, normally 10 mm.

The incidence of optic neuropathy in older studies within 5 years following conventional fractionated radiation therapy has been estimated 5–50 % for a total dose of 50 or 65 Gy delivered in 1.8–2.0 Gy/fraction (Emami et al. 1991). Actually, radiotherapy techniques used are fractionated stereotactic radiotherapy and single fraction radiosugery, most frequently with gamma knife (GKRS).

6.2.1 Fractionated Stereotactic Radiotherapy

Fractionated stereotactic radiotherapy (FSRT) delivers conventionally fractionated radiation with some degree of precision, and it has been suggested to provide increased tumor control with low toxicity. It involves the use of computed tomography and/or magnetic resonance imaging for treatment planning. The delivery of radiation is more localized than that achieved with conventional radiotherapy. It has been reported (Minniti et al. 2007) that fractionated stereotactic radiotherapy has a free survival rate higher than excision, both complete and partial.

This treatment is still susceptible to several complications including vasculitis, neuropsychological changes, worsening of visual symptoms, and, rarely, an increased occurrence of secondary tumor (Albright et al. 2005)

Stereotactic radiotherapy of small residual or recurrent craniopharyngioma may shrink tumor in approximately 58 % of patients at a mean time of 8.5 months Chiou et al. (2001) or may be used as primary treatment in small tumors where the patient is not a good surgical candidate Chung et al. (2000).

6.2.2 Radiosurgery

Stereotactic radiosurgery (SRS) is a distinct discipline that utilizes externally generated ionizing radiation to inactivate or eradicate defined target(s) in the head without the need to make an incision. The target is defined by high-resolution stereotactic imaging. To assure quality of patient care, the procedure involves a multidisciplinary team consisting of a neurosurgeon, radiation oncologist, and medical physicist. Stereotactic radiosurgery typically is performed in a single session, using a rigidly attached stereotactic guiding device, other immobilization technology, and/or a stereotactic image-guidance system. It can also be performed in a limited number of sessions, up to a maximum of five. Technologies that are used to perform SRS include linear accelerators, particle beam accelerators, and multisource Cobalt 60 units. In order to enhance precision, various devices may incorporate robotics and real-time imaging (Barnett et al. 2007).

The basis of gamma knife radiosurgery (GKRS) is stereotactic MR or CT-based planning aiming to deliver a single fraction of radiation with a sharp, steep dose falloff. The Leksell G stereotactic frame, although a little more invasive than the traditional RT mask, allows a superior degree of patient immobilization and planning precision.

Pretreatment evaluation of patients for GKRS includes systemic endocrine studies and neuro-ophthalmologic evaluation including visual field testing and visual acuity. The frame fixation is performed under mild sedation and local anesthesia. Pediatric patients are given general anesthesia for frame placement and during the whole treatment. The patient is then moved to MR suite, where noncontrast-enhanced and contrast-enhanced sequences are performed. A combination of T1-T2 sequences in axial and coronal planes are acquired as well as volumetric postcontrast 3D heavily T2W and T1 SFPGR.

This radiological protocol allows to well discriminate neural structures such as the stalk, the residual pituitary gland, the optic nerves, and the chiasm and to define tumor contour from postsurgical alterations.

The choice of radiosurgical dose for craniopharyngiomas should include the evaluation of the sensibility to radiation of the lesion and of surrounding structure and the volume of both these structures. Voluminous tumors are usually treated using conventional radiation therapy, 45 Gy delivered at 1.8–2 Gy/day fraction. The correspondence of BED of different fractionation schedules, single fraction, hypo-fractionation (3–5 fractions), or conventional fractionation is calculated using the linear quadratic model. The decision to use a single fraction or a 3–5 fraction radio-surgical schedule is based on the different sensibility to radiation of the craniopha-ryngiomas and the optic pathways in order to avoid optic neuropathy. The relative sensibility of tumor and sensitive structures is expressed by the α/β ratio derived from the linear quadratic model. In recent reviews, the traditional restrictions to 8–10 Gy to optic apparatus have been raised to 12 Gy (Pollock et al. 2014). Other cranial nerves lying within the cavernous sinus are considered to be more radiore-sistant than the optic nerves, and they can tolerate up to 15 Gy of marginal dose with no significant rate of damage.

To prevent statistically significant side effects, we usually subministrate to optic nerves under 10–12 Gy of marginal dose. Stalk is not always spared, but it must be kept under consideration that usually the patient is panhypopituitaric. Ulfarsson et al. (2002) noted that 2 patients with postradiosurgical endocrine dysfunction had received marginal doses of 15 Gy.

Much of what we know about the tolerance of normal brain structures came from studies using conventional radiation therapy and single fraction radiosur-gery. Multisession radiation allows sublethal injury to normal tissue, which can repopulate between fractions; other advantages include achieving higher tumor cell death by reoxygenation of hypoxic cells and reassortment of cells into sensi-tive phases of the cell cycle. The exact α/β ratio of craniopharyngiomas is unknown, but others have used a ratio of 2. By assuming an α/β ratio of 2, we can calculate that a radiation schedule of 25 Gy in 5 sessions estimates a singledose equivalent of 12.3 Gy, a dose that approaches our intended target. However, with an estimate of α/β ratio for craniopharyngiomas of 2 Gy (Varlotto et al. 2002), and with the reported results of tumor growth control with single doses between 9 and 12 Gy, the advantage of hypofractionation radiosurgery is questionable if a small volume of the optic pathways is exposed to doses not exceeding 12 Gy.

Several authors have reported that a therapeutic effect in craniopharyngiomas is seen with a marginal dose of 6 Gy, but the optimal dose, while not definitive, prob-ably lies between 9 and 12 Gy. Few works have presented GKRS and its results in treating craniopharyngioma, and fewer have a statistical relevancy due to little num-ber of patients. GKRS is in the majority of cases a second-line therapy, utilized to treat tumor remnants to prevent tumor recurrence or to treat a recurrent craniopha-ryngioma (Table 6.1).

Compared with surgery, GKRS is associated with relatively few complications, avoiding the immediate complications of resection as well as some of the long-term problems associated with fractionated radiotherapy. Possible complications of GKRS include hypothalamic dysfunction resulting in changes in sleep and appetite, endocrine changes, visual defects, radiation necrosis, and malignant radio-induced

Table 6.1 Results of radiosurgery treatment in patients with craniopharyngiomas

| Authors and year | No. | Mean age in years (no. of patients) | Prior resection | Intercavitary isotope TX | | Intercavitary bleomycin TX | | Mean FU (years) | Mean margin dose (Gy) | Mean TV (ml) | Tumor control rate (%) | | | | Further treatment (%) | | Morbidity rate (%) | Mortality rate (%) |
				Pre GKS	Post GKS	Pre GKS	Post GKS				Solid	Cystic	Mixed	Total	Radiation	Resection		
Lee CC et al. (2014)	137	30	69	1.5	NA	2.1	0.8	4.4	12.0	5500	73	74	66	69	27	27	11.7	9.4
Jeon et al. (2011)	13	34	100	NA	NA	NA	NA	4.8	11.0	2000	NA	NA	NA	62	NA	NA	10	10
Xu et al. (2011)	37	36	76	27	0	0	0	4.2	14.5	1600	NA	NA	NA	68	0	8	19	24
Yomo et al. (2009)	18	36	100	NA	NA	NA	NA	2.2	11.5	3500	100	67	100	94	0	0	0	0
Nirajan et al. (2010)	46	24	94	0	0	0	0	5.2	13.0	1000	78	100	59	68	11	22	17.4	2.9
Kobayashi et al. (2012)	98	<15 (38) >15 (60)	100	0	0	3	0	5.5	11.5	3500	93	79	61	80	14	1	6	5
Albright et al. (2005)	5	13	0	80	0	0	0	2.4	NA	6500	–	–	80	80	0	0	0	0
Barua et al. (2003)	7	NA	100	NA	NA	NA	NA	4.2	14.2	NA	NA	NA	NA	100	NA	NA	71	0

(continued)

Table 6.1 (continued)

Authors and year	No.	Mean age in years (no. of patients)	Prior resection	Intercavitary isotope TX		Intercavitary bleomycin TX		Mean FU (years)	Mean margin dose (Gy)	Mean TV (ml)	Tumor control rate (%)				Further treatment (%)		Morbidity rate (%)	Mortality rate (%)
				Pre GKS	Post GKS	Pre GKS	Post GKS				Solid	Cystic	Mixed	Total	Radiation	Resection		
Amendola et al. (2003)	14	12	86	8	0	0	0	3.3	14.0	3700	NA	NA	NA	86	14	0	0	0
Ulfarsson et al. (2002)	21	<15 (11) >15 (10)	56	19	23	NA	0	1.1	5.0	8000	57	100	21	36	14	0	19	0
Isaac et al. (2001)	31	32	74	6.5	0	0	3	3.0	12.2	8900	100	100	75	87	10	3	3	0
Chiou et al. (2001)	10	15	50	30	10	0	0	5.7	16.4	1700	100	–	38	58	0	10	10	0
Yu et al. (2000)	46	39	61	72	6.5	0	0	1.3	8–18(*)	13,500	90	–	86	89	0	0	0	0
Mokry et al. (1999)	23	31	39	0	0	43	4	2.0	8–10(*)	7000	–	74	–	74	13	4	0	0
Prasad et al. (1995)	9	38	67	44	11	0	0	NA	12.9	10,000	100	–	50	63	0	22	0	0

*Mean not given

Modified from Lee CC et al. (2014)

lesions such as anaplastic meningioma. Complications resulting from GKRS vary depending on patient age, tumor size, and radiation doses. However, several authors have found that GKRS provides excellent tumor control with minimal or no postoperative morbidity or mortality. In a recent review of radiosurgical series (Iannalfi et al. 2013), the mean morbidity rate was 4 %, which was considerably lower than the incidence of complications associated with resection and alternative forms of radiotherapy. Mortality was virtually absent: only Kobayashi et al. (2012) reported one case of death in his series. In a study of residual or recurrent craniopharyngiomas treated with GKRS, Chiou et al. (2001) reported visual deterioration in a single patient (10 %). Favorable quality of life outcome was most frequently demonstrated in patients with tumors that decreased in size following GKRS. Tumor regression after either initial or adjuvant GKRS has been shown in some patients with craniopharyngiomas. In a study of 5 pediatric patients, GKRS was the primary treatment for the solid portion of mixed tumors after intracavitary irradiation, which was used to treat the cystic portion, two patients experienced tumor regression, and three experienced tumor stability. Some studies exhibited higher control rates in cases of single-type tumors (solid or cystic) than in mixed-type tumors. These results are consistent with the findings of Chung et al. (2000) who found that single-type tumors, either cystic or solid, responded more effectively than mixed-type tumors of a smaller volume.

Poor quality of life outcomes after GKRS are associated with tumor progression. Larger tumor volume and multicystic tumors were predictive of poor outcome. The best outcomes were seen in patients with monocystic tumors treated with stereotactic drainage, intracavitary irradiation, or bleomycin, followed by GKRS. Ulfarsson et al. (2002) and Kobayashi et al. (2012) found that tumor progression after GKRS tended to be a function of enlargement of the cystic rather than the solid component of the tumor. It has been suggested that tumors with large cysts treated with intracavitary irradiation may benefit from GKRS after cyst size decreases. Solid-type tumors and the solid portions of mixed-type tumors are less responsive than cystic tumors to intracavitary irradiation. Prasad et al. (1995) have recommended that mixed-type tumors should be treated with a combination of radioisotype instillation and GKRS. The combined treatment of both GKRS and intracavitary irradiation has been advocated as a primary therapy for mixed cystic/ solid tumors.

Risk associated with GKRS is elevated when a large cystic volume increases the volume of the target or if there is tumor strict adherence to radiosensitive structures such as optic pathways. A multimodality treatment in such cases is useful, because large cystic or mixed-type tumors can be reduced through cyst aspiration, either in microsurgery or by an endoscopic procedure if the cystic portion lies in proximity to ventricles. Such volume reduction may reduce the risk of radiation-induced injury and allow more effective targeting of the solid portion of the tumor. In addition, an immediate improvement in a patient's condition can occur following aspiration of a cystic-type tumor, as compression of critical neural structures is relieved (Figs. 6.1 and 6.2)

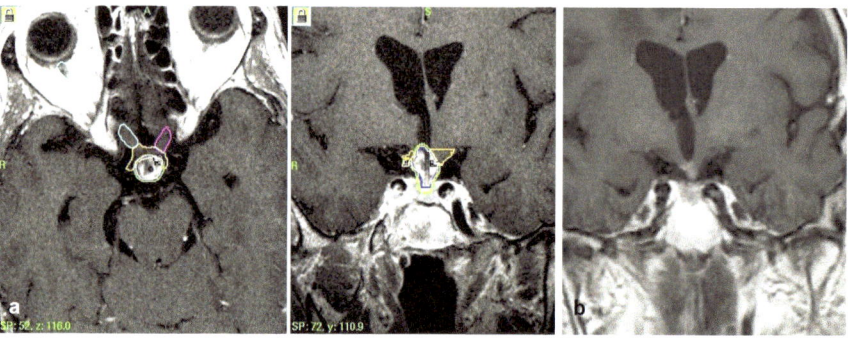

Fig. 6.1 (**a**) An example of a multimodal treatment strategy for a craniopharyngioma. This 55-year-old patient has been submitted to cyst aspiration: a ventricular catheter was left in place. The solid portion of the tumor was then treated with GKRS. Optic pathways have been carefully outlined and the marginal dose to tumor lowered to 11 Gy in order to avoid risk of optic neuropathy. (**b**) Four years follow-up: no tumor recurrence is seen; vision fields are unchanged

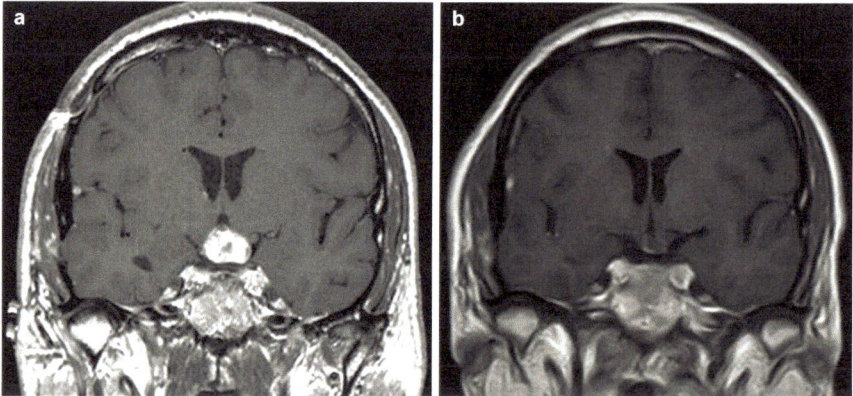

Fig. 6.2 (**a**) Postoperative residual craniopharyngioma with a cystic component treated with GKRS (12 Gy marginal dose). (**b**) 5-year follow-up: there is a marked tumor reduction. Visual acuity was stable

Conclusions

Gamma knife radiosurgery provides reasonable benefit-to-risk profile in the treatment of craniopharyngioma. In comparison to craniopharyngioma treated with resection alone, GKRS appears to be associated with a decreased rate of morbidity and mortality. Considering great precision in tumor targeting and steep fall of the irradiation dose, GKRS may also be associated with fewer complications than other forms of radiation delivery. It can be used to treat residual or recurrent craniopharyngiomas after excision; it can also be used as an initial treatment option in selected patients.

References

Albright AL, Hadjipanayis CG, Lunsford LD et al (2005) Individualized treatment of pediatric craniopharyngiomas. Childs Nerv Syst 21(8–9):649–654

Amendola BE1, Wolf A, Coy SR, Amendola MA (2003) Role of radiosurgery in craniopharyngiomas: a preliminary report. Med Pediatr Oncol 41(2):123–127

Barnett GH, Linskey ME, Adler JR et al (2007) American Association of Neurological Surgeons; Congress of Neurological Surgeons Washington Committee Stereotactic Radiosurgery Task Force. Stereotactic radiosurgery – an organized neurosurgery-sanctioned definition. Neurosurgery 106:1–5

Barua KK, Ehara K, Kohmura E, Tamaki N (2003) Treatment of recurrent craniopharyngiomas. Kobe J Med Sci 49(5-6):123–132

Chiou SM, Lunsford LD, Niranjan A et al (2001) Stereotactic radiosurgery of residual or recurrent craniopharyngioma, after surgery, with or without radiation therapy. Neuro Oncol 3:159–166

Chung WY, Pan DH, Shiau CY, Guo WY et al (2000) Gamma knife radiosurgery for craniopharyngiomas. J Neurosurg 93:47–56

Clark AJ, Cage TA, Aranda D et al (2013) A systematic review of the results of surgery and radiotherapy on tumor control for pediatric craniopharyngioma. Childs Nerv Syst 29(2):231–238

Cushing H (1932) Intracranial tumors. Notes upon a series of two thousand verified cases with surgical-mortality percentages pertaining thereto. Charles, Springfield

Di Pinto M, Conklin HM, Li C et al (2010) Learning and memory following conformal radiation therapy for pediatric craniopharyngioma and low-grade glioma. Int J Radiat Oncol Biol Phys 84(3):e363–e369

Emami B, Lyman J, Brown A et al (1991) Tolerance of normal tissue to therapeutic irradiation. Int J Radiat Oncol Biol Phys 21(1):109–122

Hargrave DR (2006) Does chemotherapy have a role in the management of craniopharyngioma? J Pediatr Endocrinol Metab 19(Suppl):407–412

Iannalfi A, Fragkandrea I, Brock J et al (2013) Radiotherapy in craniopharyngiomas. Clin Oncol (R Coll Radiol) 25(11):654–667

Isaac MA, Hahn SS, Kim JA, Bogart JA, Chung CT (2001) Management of craniopharyngioma. Cancer J 7(6):516–520

Jeon C, Kim S, Shin HJ, Nam DH (2011) The therapeutic efficacy of fractionated radiotherapy and gamma-knife radiosurgery for craniopharyngiomas. J Clin Neurosci 18(12):1621–1625

Karavitaki N, Cudlip S, Adams CB et al (2006) Craniopharyngiomas. Endocr Rev 27:371–397

Kobayashi T, Mori Y, Tsugawa T et al (2012) Prognostic factors for tumor recurrence after gamma knife radiosurgery of partially resected and recurrent craniopharyngiomas. Nagoya J Med Sci 74:141–147

Lee CC, Yang HC, Chen CJ et al (2014) Gamma Knife surgery for craniopharyngioma: report on a 20-year experience. J Neurosurg 121(Suppl 2):167–178

Liubinas SV, Munshey AS, Kaye A (2011) Management of recurrent craniopharyngioma. J Clin Neurosci 18:451–457

Lopez-Serna R, Gomez-Amadorv JL (2012) Treatment of craniopharyngioma in adults: systematic analysis of a 25-year experience. Arch Med Res 43:347–355

Minniti G, Saran F, Traish D et al (2007) Fractionated stereotactic conformal radiotherapy following conservative surgery in the control of craniopharyngiomas. Radiother Oncol 82:90–95

Mokry M (1999) Craniopharyngiomas: A six year experience with Gamma Knife radiosurgery. Stereotact Funct Neurosurg 72(Suppl 1):140–149

Mortini P, Losa M, Pozzobon G et al (2011) Neurosurgical treatment of craniopharyngioma in adults and children: early and long-term results in a large case series. J Neurosurg 114:1350–1359

Müller HL, Gebhardt U, Schröder S et al (2010) Analyses of treatment variables for patients with childhood craniopharyngioma – results of the multicenter prospective trial KRANIOPHARYNGEOM 2000 after three years of follow-up. Horm Res Paediatr 73:175e180

Niranjan A, Kano H, Mathieu D, Kondziolka D, Flickinger JC, Lunsford LD (2010) Radiosurgery for craniopharyngioma. Int J Radiat Oncol Biol Phys 78(1):64–71

Pollock BE, Link MJ, Leavitt JA et al (2014) Dose-volume analysis of radiation-induced optic neuropathy after single-fraction stereotactic radiosurgery. Neurosurgery 75(4):456–460

Prasad D, Steiner M, Steiner L (1995) Gamma knife surgery for craniopharyngioma. Acta Neurochir (Wien) 134:167–176

Rickert CH, Paulus W (2001) Epidemiology of central nervous systemtumors in childhood and adolescence based on the new WHO classification. Childs Nerv Syst 17(9):503–511

Rodriguez F, Scheithaur BW, Tsunoda S et al (2007) The spectrum of malignancy in craniopharyngioma. Am J Surg Pathol 31(7):1020–1027

Samii M, Tatagiba M (1997) Surgical management of craniopharyngiomas:a review. Neurol Med Chir (Tokyo) 37(2):141–149

Ulfarsson E, Lindquist C, Roberts M et al (2002) Gamma knife radiosurgery for craniopharyngiomas: long-term results in the first Swedish patients. J Neurosurg 97(5 Suppl):613–622

Varlotto JM, Flickinger JC, Kondziolka D et al (2002) External beam irradiation of craniopharyngiomas: longterm analysis of tumor control and morbidity. Int J Radiat Oncol Biol Phys 54:492–499

Xu Z, Yen CP, Schlesinger D, Sheehan J (2011) Outcomes of Gamma Knife surgery for craniopharyngiomas. J Neurooncol 104(1):305–313

Yomo S, Hayashi M, Chernov M (2009) Stereotactic radiosurgery of residual or recurrent craniopharyngioma: new treatment concept using Leksell gamma knife model C with automatic positioning system. Stereotact Funct Neurosurg 87(6):360–367

Yu X, Liu Z, Li S (2000) Combined treatment with stereotactic intracavitary irradiation and gamma knife surgery for craniopharyngiomas. Stereotact Funct Neurosurg 75(2-3):117–122

Endocrine Consequences: Diagnostic Workout and Treatment

7

Claudia Giavoli

Abstract

Craniopharyngiomas are in general slowly growing tumors and symptoms may develop gradually. The most common presenting clinical symptoms are visual field deficits and signs of hypopituitarism that may be present at diagnosis but also after surgery. In this chapter, clinical presentation, diagnosis, and treatment of pituitary hormone deficiencies will be reviewed.

Craniopharyngiomas are in general slowly growing tumors and symptoms may develop gradually as reflected by the observation that a delay of 1–2 years between symptom onset and diagnosis is often present (Garnettet et al. 2007). The most common presenting clinical symptoms are visual field deficits and signs of hypopituitarism such as impaired growth and puberty arrest (in children) and menstrual irregularities, impaired sexual function, and poor energy (in adults) (Karavitaki et al. 2005). In children, at presentation growth hormone deficiency is the most common pituitary deficit (up to 100 % of patients), followed by ACTH (25 % of patients) and TSH (up to 25 % of patients) deficiency. In adults, growth hormone deficiency is reported in 80–90 % of cases, gonadotropin deficiency in present in 70 % of patients, followed by ACTH deficiency (up to 40 % of patients) and TSH deficiency (40 % of patients) (Karavitaki et al. 2005, 2006a, b; Muller 2014).

Surgery is the treatment of choice of craniopharyngiomas and contrary to what is reported in pituitary adenomas, no reversal of preexisting pituitary hormone deficiencies after surgical intervention have been reported (Karavitaki et al. 2006a, b). According to published series, postsurgical hypopituitarism is diagnosed in the majority of patients. In particular, GH deficiency is reported in 90–100 % of

C. Giavoli, MD
Unit of Endocrinology and Metabolic Diseases, Fondazione IRCCS Cà Granda Ospedale Maggiore Policlinico, Via F. Sforza 35, Milan 10122, Italy
e-mail: claudiagiavoli@yahoo.it

© Springer International Publishing Switzerland 2016
A. Lania et al. (eds.), *Diagnosis and Management of Craniopharyngiomas: Key Current Topics*, DOI 10.1007/978-3-319-22297-4_7

patients, gonadotropin deficiency is diagnosed in 80–95 % of patients, central hypoadrenalism is present in 50–88 % of patients, and central hypothyroidism is reported in 40–95 % of cases (Karavitaki et al. 2006a, b; Muller 2014).

7.1 GH Deficiency

Growth hormone deficiency (GHD) in adults has been found to be associated to an increased morbidity and mortality secondary to the deleterious effects of GHD on several cardiovascular risk factors (Gazzaruso et al. 2014). Untreated adults with GHD show an increase of visceral adipose tissue associated to a reduction in lean body mass; these alterations in body composition lead to the development of the metabolic syndrome (Attanasio et al. 2010). In this respect, the increase in visceral adiposity leads to insulin resistance. GHD patients present an increase in total and LDL cholesterol and apolipoprotein B levels due to an impaired lipid clearance (Abdu et al. 2001; Gazzaruso et al. 2014). Hypertension is a common feature of severe GH deficiency, and echocardiography studies demonstrate a reduction in left ventricular mass and function that is prevalent in adults with childhood-onset GH deficiency (Attanasio et al. 2010; Lombardi et al. 2012). Adult GHD patients show also a slight reduction in BMD, the severity of this BMD impairment being possibly related to the age at onset of GHD (Kaufman et al. 1992; Holmes et al. 1994). Despite this slight reduction in BMD, adult patients with GHD are characterized by a significant increase in fracture rate (Wuster et al. 2001). Finally, GHD is associated to a reduced quality of life. In particular, adult GHD patients complain depressed mood, anxiety, social isolation, and deficits in memory and concentration (Moock et al. 2009) (Table 7.1).

Children typically fall in the growth curves and growth velocity becomes abnormal. Notably, slow growth compared with other children of the same age is the first sign of GHD, present before the onset of short stature. Thus, it is important to look at the child's growth charts, also in relation to the target height. Delayed puberty, also due to concomitant gonadotropins deficiency, may be present along with delayed bone age.

Table 7.1 Clinical manifestations of GHD in adults

⇑ Visceral adipose tissue
⇓ Lean body mass
⇓ Skeletal muscle strength and exercise performance
⇓ BMD ⇑ risk of fracture
Atherogenic lipid profile
Thin, dry skin
Impaired quality of life (e.g., fatigue, depression, anxiety, impaired sleep, and social isolation)

7.1.1 Diagnosis

Since signs and symptoms of GHD in adults are nonspecific, the diagnosis requires biochemical testing. Due to the episodic pattern of GH secretion, low random GH levels are not diagnostic (Molitch et al. 2011). Similarly, IGF-1 measurement may be not specific and sensitive enough to diagnose a GHD since there is a significant overlap in IGF-1 levels between normal subjects and those with GHD (Molitch et al. 2011; Biller et al. 2002). Moreover, IGF-1 levels may be reduced in conditions other than GHD. In fact, fasting, oral estrogens, liver diseases, and catabolic conditions are characterized by low circulating IGF-1. Therefore, provocative tests are required to identify a patient with GHD (Molitch et al. 2011) (Table 7.2).

Insulin tolerance test (ITT, 0.1 units/kg IV regular insulin; measure glucose and GH at baseline and every 30 min for 3 h) is recommended as the gold standard among provocative tests for GHD, a GH less than 3 mcg/ml (adults) and less than 10 mcg/ml (children) being diagnostic for GH deficiency (Molitch et al. 2011). ITT requires blood glucose levels of <40 mg/dl (<2.2 mmol/l) to be diagnostic, and it is contraindicated in patients affected by ischemic heart disease, in the elderly, and in epileptics.

Nowadays, the arginine plus GHRH stimulation test (GHRH 1 μg/kg plus arginine 0.5 g/kg over 30 min; measure GH at baseline and every 30 min for 3 h) has been validated, and it is considered an acceptable alternative to ITT (Molitch et al. 2011; Aimaretti et al. 1998). Contrary to ITT, it is generally free of adverse effects or contraindications. Compared to other stimulation tests, cutoff values used to diagnose GH deficiency with arginine plus GHRH are strongly dependent on BMI (Corneli et al. 2005). In particular, GHD is diagnosed if GH peak is less than 11 mcg/l, 8 mcg/l, and 4 mcg/l and if BMI is <25, between 25 and 30, and >30 kg/m^2, respectively (Corneli et al. 2005). It is worth noting that, because GHRH directly stimulates the pituitary, it can give a falsely normal GH response in patients with GHD of hypothalamic origin (Darzy et al. 2003).

To diagnose GHD in children, many alternative stimuli are now currently used, such as clonidine, arginine, L-dopa, and glucagon (Molitch et al. 2011). This last test is particularly useful in pediatric age, since it allows simultaneous evaluation of

Table 7.2 Testing in GHD patients

	Test	Cutoff
Children		
	Insulin tolerance test (ITT)	10 mcg/l
	Clonidine	10 mcg/l
	Arginine	10 mcg/l
	Glucagon	10 mcg/l
Adults		
	Insulin tolerance test (ITT)	3 mcg/l
	Arginine + GHRH	BMI <25: 11 mcg/l
		BMI ≥25 <30: 8 mcg/l
		BMI ≥30: 4 mcg/l

GH and adrenal axis as ITT, but with less adverse effects. Combined stimuli such as GHRH + arginine or GHRH + pyridostigmine can also be used. The cutoff is a GH peak less than 20 ng/ml for combined tests and less than 10 ng/ml for other ones though the cut-off has been lowered to 8 μg/L, at least in Italy, as proposed by the new note 39 of the Italian Medicine Agency (AIFA). In the presence of multiple pituitary deficiency, a single test is sufficient for the diagnosis of GHD in children if the test is a combined one, while two pathological tests are necessary for diagnosis of GHD for all the other tests.

Finally, presence of deficiencies in three or more pituitary axes strongly suggests the presence of GHD thus suggesting that in these conditions provocative testing is optional (Molitch et al. 2011; Hartman et al. 2002).

7.1.2 Treatment

GH deficiency replacement therapy in adults should be individualized and not based on body weight (Molitch et al. 2011; Hoffman et al. 2004). It is advisable to start with low daily doses of recombinant human GH (0.2 mg SC at bedtime) to be gradually increased on the basis of IGF-I levels and the possible appearance of side effects and the clinical response (i.e., body composition, exercise capacity, psychological well-being, bone density, and cardiovascular risk factors modifications) (Molitch et al. 2011). In patients <30 years of age, it is reasonable to start with higher doses. Conversely, patients older than 60 years of age should start with doses <0.2–0.4 mg per day (Molitch et al. 2011). Typically, higher doses are required in women with normal gonadal function or taking oral estrogen-progestin or in post-menopausal women treated with estrogen replacement therapy (Burman et al. 1997; Molitch et al. 2011). IGF-I circulating levels should be maintained around the median or in the upper half of the normal range for age and should be checked every 1–2 months until the maintenance dose has been reached and then every 6 months (Molitch et al. 2011) (Table 7.3).

At the beginning of GH replacement therapy, possible adverse events are related to fluid retention induced by GH. In particular, up to 20 % of adult patients may

Table 7.3 Follow-up of adult GHD patients during GH replacement therapy

Parameter	Frequency
IGF-1	Every 4–8 weeks and the every 6 weeks
Glucose profile	Annually
Lipid profile	Annually
ACTH stimulation test	At baseline and 4 weeks after GH starting if symptoms suggest hypoadrenalism
Blood pressure, weight, waist circumference, and BMI	Annually
Dexa	Every 2 years if basal Dexa shows osteopenia or osteoporosis
Quality of life	Annually

complain of edema, arthralgias, myalgias, paresthesias, and carpal tunnel syndrome; these side effects disappear with dose reduction (Molitch et al. 2011); these adverse events are relatively more frequent in obese, elderly, and female patients. Interestingly, GH replacement therapy does not induce a significant growth of craniopharyngiomas and pituitary adenomas as demonstrated by large observational studies both in adults and children (Karavitaki et al. 2006a, b).

During GH replacement therapy, both thyroid and adrenal function should be carefully evaluated (Molitch et al. 2011). In fact, in nearly 50 % of euthyroid patients at baseline, FT4 levels dramatically fall into the hypothyroid range during GH treatment, thus requiring the beginning of L-thyroxine replacement therapy (Porretti et al. 2002). Similarly, up to 20 % of patients treated for central hypothyroidism need an increase in L-thyroxine doses to normalize FT4 during GH treatment (Porretti et al. 2002). To explain these findings, it has been hypothesized that IGF-1 normalization induces both an increase of T4 to T3 peripheral conversion and the acceleration of thyroid hormones' metabolic clearance. GH replacement therapy may also affect the hypothalamus-pituitary-adrenal axis function. In fact, GH replacement therapy may unmask a central hypoadrenalism; this condition being the consequence of the inhibitory effect of GH on 11β-hydroxy steroid dehydrogenase type 1 activity thus leads to a reduced conversion of cortone to cortisol (Consensus 2000).

In children, treatment goal is the normalization of growth velocity, in order to promote the achievement of a normal stature, also according to target height (Consensus 2000). Along with the main effect on longitudinal growth, GH replacement is also able to restore normal body composition, to promote the attainment of a normal peak bone mass, and to support adequate growth and development of all organs. Recommended dose ranges from 0.025 to 0.035 mg/kg/day, varying according to age and pubertal stages (Consensus 2000). Therapy should be started as soon as possible to maximize its effect, but stability of the disease should be documented. The first year of therapy is characterized by a dramatic increase in growth velocity (i.e., catch-up growth), in which a child's height tends to reach its physiological curve; subsequently growth rate slowly returns to normal values for sex and age. The efficacy of GH therapy is documented in both normalization of growth velocity and of IGF-I levels; the latter used also as a safety tool to avoid overtreatment. The therapy should be continued till growth velocity falls under 2 cm/year and hand and wrist radiography documents closure of epiphyseal cartilages. In children, possible adverse effects of GH therapy, which are indeed not common, are headache, arthralgias, alteration of glucose metabolism, and epiphysiolysis of femoral head. Intracranial hypertension is extremely rare.

7.2 Central Hypogonadism

The clinical picture of the hypogonadism depends on the time of manifestation of the disorder (Table 7.4). When the onset of hypogonadism takes place around pubertal period, the main symptom, both in boys and in girls, is lack or arrest of pubertal development.

Table 7.4 Age-dependent clinical features of hypogonadism in male

	Prepubertal onset	Adult onset
Larynx	High-pitched voice	No change of voice
Body proportions	Eunuchoid habitus	No changes
Skin	Absent sebum production, no acne, pallor, skin wrinkling	
Muscles	Underdeveloped	Atrophy
Penis	Infantile	Normal size
Testes	Possibly maldescended testes, small volume	Reduced volume
Libido and potency	Absent	Erectile dysfunction

Boys affected by hypogonadism are clinically characterized by micropenis, small testis size (less than 2 ml), and reduced virilization. The absence of testosterone is associated to a delayed epiphyseal closure, thus leading to the appearance of eunuchoid habitus (i.e., arm span exceeding body length and legs becoming longer than the trunk). Eunuchoidism is also characterized by poor muscle mass development (especially in the shoulders and chest) and prepubertal fat distribution (i.e., the face, chest, and hips) (Rogol 2005; Silveira and Latronico 2013). In girls lack of estrogen production leads to impaired secondary sexual development and primary amenorrhea (Silveira and Latronico 2013).

Male adults most commonly present with sexual dysfunction (diminished libido, reduced spontaneous and sexually evoked erections, and erectile dysfunction), gynecomastia and infertility, and impaired spermatogenesis (i.e., oligozoospermia or azoospermia) (Basaria 2014). In patients with severe and long-standing hypogonadism, loss of androgen-dependent hair (i.e., facial hairs) as well as loss of axillary and pubic hair may be observed (Hayes et al. 1998). Since testosterone, via estradiol, is important in the maintenance of bone mass, osteopenia or osteoporosis may be present in adult males with hypogonadism (Irwig 2013; Basaria 2014). Long-standing testosterone deficiency leads to reduced muscle mass and strength, thus leading to weakness and reduced physical performance (Smith et al. 2002; Finkelstein et al. 2013; Basaria 2014). This reduction in lean mass may be associated to an increase in central body fat accumulation (Smith et al. 2002; Finkelstein et al. 2013). Skin changes and reduced sebum production cause fine facial wrinkling particularly on the lateral corners of the orbits and mouth. Signs of vasomotor instability such as hot flushes and sweats may be reported, mainly when testosterone deficiency occurs rapidly; these symptoms are similar to those experienced by menopausal women. Men with chronic low testosterone concentrations often complain of diminished vitality, depressed mood, increased sleepiness, or poor concentration and memory (Basaria 2014). Men with severe androgen deficiency may have a mild normocytic, normochromic anemia. Though testis size may be small in most men with acquired adult hypogonadism, testis size is normal to slightly reduced (Basaria 2014).

In adult premenopausal female, the loss of ovarian function is manifested with oligomenorrhea or amenorrhea, infertility, and symptoms of hypoestrogenism such as decreased vaginal discharge, dyspareunia, decreased libido, loss of pubic and axillary hair, breast atrophy, and osteoporosis (Hayes et al. 1998; Misra 2012). In patients with a severe hypogonadism, signs of vasomotor instability such as hot flushes and sweats may be reported. In postmenopausal women, however, hypogonadism is not associated to any specific sign or symptom.

7.2.1 Diagnosis

Hormonal evaluation shows normal/low gonadotropin levels along with low sex steroids levels (Silveira and Latronico 2013). Biochemical diagnosis of hypogonadism may be difficult in infancy, when concentrations of sex steroids and gonadotropins are physiologically low. Although serum LH and FSH levels are pulsatile, testing can be valuable. Puberty begins when GnRH secretion increases and serum LH rises disproportionately to FSH. Serum LH levels are usually below 0.3 mIU/ml before puberty and range from 2 to 12 mIU/ml during later stages of puberty and into adulthood. Serum FSH levels are usually <3 mIU/ml before puberty and fluctuate between 5 and 10 mIU/ml during the second half of puberty and into adulthood. Dynamic testing with GnRH is not necessary if the hormonal evaluation shows hypopituitarism. Anyway, it usually shows a prepubertal response of gonadotropins, with FSH increase greater than the one of LH (Dunkel and Quinton 2014).

In adult males, serum testosterone is the laboratory value most important for both diagnosing hypogonadism and monitoring testosterone substitution therapy (Rosner et al. 2007; Bhasin et al. 2010). When interpreting testosterone values, it is necessary to consider that morning serum concentrations are approximately 20–40 % higher than evening values. Moreover, testosterone is bound to sex hormone-binding globulin (SHBG), only approximately 2 % of testosterone being unbound and as circulating free testosterone available for biological activity (Rosner et al. 2007). Since direct free testosterone measurement is still inaccurate and therefore not reccomended, a standardized formula has proved to be a simple and reliable method for estimating testosterone bioactivity (Rosner et al. 2007; Bhasin et al. 2010). Finally, physical exercise, chronic diseases, stress, anesthesia, drugs, and certain medications may affect circulating testosterone levels (Rosner et al. 2007).

Considering all these factors, normal serum testosterone concentration in the adult male lies between 12 and 40 nmol/l during the first half of the day. Concentrations below 8 nmol/l are certainly pathological (Rosner et al. 2007). Conversely, values between 8 and 12 require the evaluation of a calculated free testosterone mainly in symptomatic patients (Bhasin et al. 2010).

7.2.2 Treatment

According to international consensus, the major goal of testosterone therapy is to replace testosterone levels at as close to physiological concentrations as is possible.

In this view, the naturally occurring testosterone molecule should be used for substitution.

7.2.2.1 Prepubertal Patients

In general, replacement therapy should induce puberty and manifestation of sexual characters; to this aim sex steroids are always used. Therapy should be started when the normal onset of puberty is expected, i.e., 13.5–14 in boys and 12.5–13 years in girls. In the hypogonadic adolescent boy, long-acting testosterone preparation is mainly used, with the starting dose of 25 mg intramuscular (IM) every 15 days or 50 mg/month during the first year, 100 mg/month during the second year, and thereafter 250 mg/month. Transdermal preparation of testosterone can also be used, though are less accepted by young boys and adolescents. In order to achieve an adequate testicular development, gonadotropins can later be used, for a period no longer than 2 years, and then later on to achieve spermatogenesis when fertility is desired (hCG 1000–2000 IU three times/week IM and rhFSH 75 IU IM 2–3 times/week) (Dunkel and Quinton 2014).

In hypogonadic girl, therapy consists in the administration of increasing dose of estrogens given orally or transdermally. The starting ethinyl estradiol dose is 0.1 mcg/kg/day, to be increased every 6 months, to induce regular pubertal development. Thereafter, sequential estroprogestative therapy is initiated to induce regular menstruation.

Adults Patients

In males, the major goal of testosterone therapy is to replace testosterone levels at as close to physiological concentrations as is possible. The choice of a single testosterone preparation should be based on several considerations such as the age of patient, patient's preferences, and possible coexistence of other illnesses (Bhasin et al. 2010).

Testosterone undecanoate is given orally, two to four capsules spread over the course of a day (80–160 mg per day) being required for substitution. The disadvantage of this testosterone preparation lies primarily in the poor predictability of individual resorption patterns. Moreover, this preparation does not mimic the physiological testosterone secretion pattern due to the short-lived peaks and troughs in serum testosterone (Basaria 2014).

Intramuscular administration of testosterone enanthate is the form most widely used in testosterone replacement therapy, the standard dose being 200–250 mg testosterone enanthate every 21–28 days. Supraphysiological serum testosterone concentrations are rapidly achieved and then gradually declined, passing the lower level of normal on about day 12. For this reason, replacement therapy requires repeated injections that induce the alternanza of supraphysiological, physiological, and infraphysiological levels. This testosterone level profile may affect general well-being, moods, and sexual activity, a condition that may be disturbing for the patient. Individual intervals are determined according to serum testosterone levels which are measured immediately before the next injection (Basaria 2014).

Testosterone undecanoate IM is characterized by a long half-life and by the absence of initial supraphysiological peaks. In males with hypogonadism, 1000 mg testosterone undecanoate are injected about four times per year. Individual intervals are determined according to serum testosterone levels which are measured immediately before the next injection (Basaria 2014).

Among the transdermal testosterone preparations so far available, testosterone gels are those more frequently used. These 1 % testosterone gels (50 mg per day) are applied in the morning (to mimic the physiological testosterone secretion profile) to the upper arm, shoulders, and abdomen and are left to dry for 5 min. During this time, no contacts with women or children should be allowed in order to prevent any possible contamination (Basaria 2014).

Testosterone replacement therapy should be regularly monitored by evaluating male hair pattern, muscle mass and strength, hemoglobin, erythrocyte count and hematocrit, lipid profile, PSA levels and prostate volume, and bone mass. Finally, testosterone replacement therapy is contraindicated in patients with breast or prostate cancer, in patients with hematocrit above 50 %, untreated severe obstructive sleep apnea, severe lower urinary tract symptoms, or uncontrolled or poorly controlled heart failure (Bhasin et al. 2010).

In adult female patients, transdermal estradiol (usually 100 mcg daily) or oral estradiol (usually 2 mg/day) are generally used (Silveira and Latronico 2013). This dose is also roughly equivalent to 1.25 mg of conjugated equine estrogen or about 10 mcg of ethinyl estradiol. The use of transdermal patch provides 17beta-estradiol, which is structurally identical to ovarian 17beta-estradiol and reduces the risk of venous thromboembolism compared with the oral route (by avoiding the first-pass effect on the liver possibly associated with an increase in clotting factors' production). Because most of these women have an intact uterus, an effective progestin regimen to fully reduce the risk of endometrial hyperplasia and carcinoma is critical. In this view, it is advisable to use 10 mg of medroxyprogesterone acetate per day for the first 10–12 calendar days of each month.

The fertility of patients with central hypogonadism can be restored through the use of GnRH or, more commonly, with the use of gonadotropins. In particular, in male gonadotropin treatment starts with the administration of 1000–2500 IU of hCG twice a week for 8–12 weeks. Subsequently, the treatment continues with the coadministration of hCG and either 75–150 IU hMG or 150 IU of recombinant FSH three times per week up to 12–18 months (Zitzmann and Nieschlag 2000; Han and Bouloux 2010). Though the total number of sperm remains below the normal range, impregnation rate reaches 50–80 % in patients with a sperm concentration of 5 million per ml (Zitzmann and Nieschlag 2000; Han and Bouloux 2010).

7.3   Central Hypoadrenalism

Central hypoadrenalism is a condition of reduced adrenal function secondary to an ACTH secretion deficiency. This condition is frequently diagnosed in patients with both pituitary and hypothalamus tumors, the highest frequency being found in patients operated on for craniopharyngiomas (Crowley et al. 2010).

Clinical manifestations of central hypoadrenalism are similar to those of Addison's disease, although sometimes less defined. Adult patients may be asymptomatic, and the disease may be diagnosed during stressful events leading to a crisis. Unlike the primary hypoadrenalism, in patients with central adrenal insufficiency electrolyte abnormalities and postural hypotension are less frequently observed. However, hyponatremia and volume expansion can occur secondary to an inappropriate increase in antidiuretic hormone secretion (SIADH). Patients with chronic central hypoadrenalism may present weakness, easy fatigability, arthralgia, myalgia, weight loss, anorexia, nausea, and sometimes vomiting (Grossman 2010; Crowley et al. 2014).

7.3.1 Diagnosis

Since the circadian peak serum cortisol usually occurs around 8.00 in the morning, very low morning cortisol levels should be diagnostic of a condition of adrenal insufficiency. In this view, according to a recent meta-analysis (Kazlauskaite et al. 2008), a morning cortisol greater than 18 mcg/dl (500 nmol/l) is considered to be predictive of a normal hypothalamus-pituitary-adrenal (HPA) axis function thus not requiring any confirmatory dynamic test. Conversely, the finding of a morning cortisol less than 3 mcg/dl (80 nmol/l) should indicate an impaired HPA axis function, and patients should be treated appropriately. However, in the presence of cortisol levels between 3 and 18 mcg/dl, dynamic tests should be performed to explore the HPA axis function (Grossman 2010; Crowley et al. 2014; Øksnes et al. 2015) (Fig. 7.1).

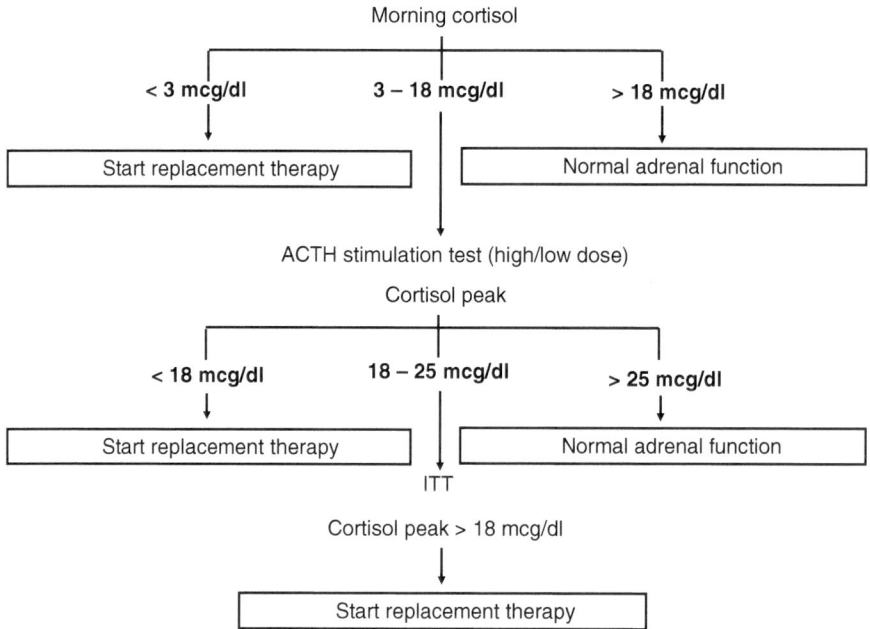

Fig. 7.1 Central hypocortisolism: diagnostic flowchart. ITT, insulin tolerance test

The ACTH stimulation test has been proved to be effective in identifying patients with central hypoadrenalism. Since a prolonged ACTH deficiency causes an adrenal cortex hypotrophy, a subnormal cortisol response to exogenous ACTH is indicative of adrenal insufficiency. Because failure of adrenal reserve in response to ACTH deficiency requires time to develop, the test should be performed at least 3–6 weeks after pituitary-hypothalamus surgery (Grossman 2010). The so-called high-dose ACTH stimulation test is performed by injecting ACTH [1–24] 0.25 mg IV. Cortisol is then measured at 0, 30, and 60 min, and hypoadrenalism is diagnosed if peak cortisol is less than 18 mcg/dl (500 nmol/l). A low-dose ACTH test (ACTH [1–24] 1 mcg IV) has been also proposed to reduce the possible false negatives due to the fact that supraphysiological doses of ACTH may overcome partial adrenal atrophy. To avoid false-positive results, the aliquot of 1 ml (1 mcg) of ACTH should be rigorously prepared. Several studies have questioned the appropriateness of 18 mcg/dl (500 nmol/l) cutoff to exclude the presence of central adrenal insufficiency, thus suggesting the opportunity to perform an insulin tolerance test (ITT) in patients having a peak cortisol between 15 and 25 mcg/dl after ACTH stimulation test (Grossman 2010; Crowley et al. 2014; Øksnes et al. 2015) (Fig. 7.1). ITT (regular insulin 0.05–0.1 U/kg IV, cortisol measured over 120 min), by inducing symptomatic and biochemical hypoglycemia, is effective to evaluate the integrity of the HPA axis. In particular, hypoadrenalism is diagnosed when cortisol does not increase above 18 mcg/dl (500 nmol/l) in the presence of a glycemia less than <40 mg/dl (<2.2 mmol/l). It is worth noting that ITT is contraindicated in elderly patients with a history of ischemic heart disease and in young children (<6 years). Finally, ITT may be used to simultaneously evaluate the integrity of the HPA axis and GH reserve. Importantly, diagnostic tests should never delay the start of glucocorticoid treatment in patients with suspected adrenal crisis. In these patients, confirmation of diagnosis by dynamic tests can be performed after clinical recovery.

7.3.2 Treatment

The aim of glucocorticoid replacement therapy is to restore normal cortisol levels mimicking the physiological circadian cortisol secretion rhythm, this condition being reached using the lowest dose of glucocorticoid (Johannsson et al. 2012). Recommended hydrocortisone doses are 15–25 mg, usually given in two to three doses per day, with 50–60 % given on awakening. In two times a day regimen, the second dose is given 6–8 h after the morning dose. In three times per day regimen, the second dose is usually given 4–6 h after the morning dose and the third dose 4–6 h after the second one. The replacement therapy regimen should be decided on the basis of patient preference and daily activity. In the treatment of central hypoadrenalism, other glucocorticoids such as prednisone (or prednisolone) and cortisone may be used (Øksnes et al. 2015). However, cortisone and prednisone may be characterized by a higher pharmacokinetic variability compared with hydrocortisone due to the fact that these compounds should be activated (to cortisol and prednisolone, respectively) by11β-hydroxysteroid dehydrogenase type 1 (Øksnes et al. 2015). Recently, a modified-release formulation of hydrocortisone (Plenadren®) characterized by an immediate release coating combined with an extended-release core has been licensed. The medication is taken on awakening in a single daily dose, and it has been demonstrated that in patients taking Plenadren 24 h, exposure of cortisol is reduced thus inducing a reduction of body weight, blood pressure, and glucose profile (Johannsson et al. 2012). However, the bioavailability of the compound is 20 % less than oral hydrocortisone, and dose adjustments are frequently required (Johannsson et al. 2009).

The dose in children is based on body surface area and usually ranges from 6 to 10 mg/m2/day, distributing the dose twice or better thrice daily. In case of stress, such as illness or surgery, hydrocortisone dose should be increased and can be administered by injection (hydrocortisone 100 mg) if vomiting or diarrhea are present (Hahner and Allolio 2009).

Contrary to what happen in patients taking GH and L-thyroxine replacement therapies, there are no reliable biochemical markers to assess the appropriateness of dose in glucocorticoid replacement treatment. In this respect, too low glucocorticoid doses increase the risk of adrenal crisis and reduce well-being, whereas glucocorticoid therapy excess is associated to complications such as osteoporosis, obesity, and impaired glucose tolerance (Øksnes et al. 2015). Dose modifications depend on clinical judgment and perception of symptoms and signs of glucocorticoid under- and over-replacement by the patient (Øksnes et al. 2015). Morning fatigue may suggest low cortisol levels, this condition being overcome by suggesting the patient to take the morning dose 30–60 min before he gets up. Difficulties falling asleep may indicate that the late dose is taken too late.

It is worth noting that in patients with multiple pituitary hormone deficiency, as frequently observed in patients with craniopharyngiomas, GH and estrogen replacement therapies may affect glucocorticoid metabolism. It has been demonstrated that IGF-1 normalization during GH replacement may unmask central hypoadrenalism by increasing cortisol clearance secondary to by11β-hydroxysteroid dehydrogenase type 1 (Giavoli et al. 2004). Higher glucocorticoid doses may be required in women receiving oral estrogens since estrogens induce cortisol-binding globulin levels.

Adrenal crisis is a life-threatening emergency; the most frequent precipitating causes being gastroenteritis and fever followed by other stressful events such as trauma, surgery, and dental procedures. In many cases, crises are the consequences of an inadequate glucocorticoid dose increase (Øksnes et al. 2015). The main clinical manifestations are abdominal symptoms such as epigastric pain, diarrhea, nausea, vomiting, and anorexia. This condition is usually associated to hypotension and severe asthenia. Laboratory tests show electrolyte alterations such as hyponatremia and hyperkalemia, normocytic normochromic anemia, neutropenia with a relative lymphocytosis, and eosinophilia. Because of dehydration and volume depletion, there is an increase in blood urea nitrogen and creatinine. Hypoglycemia, mild hypercalcemia, and a mild acidosis are also frequent. The treatment of the crisis is based on the prompt administration of hydrocortisone (100 mg IV every 6 h in the first 24 h to be gradually adjusted in relation to the clinical response) (Øksnes et al. 2015).

7.4   Central Hypothyroidism

Central hypothyroidism (CH) is an uncommon cause of hypothyroidism in both children and adults, accounting for probably less than 1–2 % of all cases of hypothyroidism. Craniopharyngioma and pituitary adenomas, particularly macroadenomas, are the most frequent cause of TSH deficiency in children and adults, respectively.

Clinical features of CH may vary depending on the severity of the thyroid impairment, number of associated hormone deficiencies, and age of the patient at the time of disease onset. The clinical picture is generally indistinguishable from that of primary hypothyroidism, except for the presence of symptoms due to hypothalamus-pituitary mass (headache, visual disturbances), and is essentially determined by the duration and extent of the lack of thyroid hormone (Lania et al. 2008). Typically, CH symptoms are milder than those of primary hypothyroidism. Adult patients with CH may present with adynamia, dry skin, drowsiness, intolerance to cold, reducing memory and attentional capacity, constipation, hoarse voice, menstrual irregularities to amenorrhea, hypercholesterolemia, hypertriglyceridemia, and anemia (Lania et al. 2008). It is worth noting that in adult patients, goiter is always absent. In children delayed growth is the most evident clinical sign (Lania et al. 2008).

7.4.1   Diagnosis

Contrary to what is usually done in primary hypothyroidism, both TSH and free T4 should be measured to correctly diagnose CH (Baloch et al. 2003). In fact, in these patients TSH is usually in the normal range or even slightly increased in patients with a prevalent hypothalamic defect thus suggesting the secretion of TSH molecules characterized by a low biological activity (Baloch et al. 2003). Accordingly, free T4 is the parameter of thyroid function characterized by the highest sensitivity and specificity for diagnosis of CH (Baloch et al. 2003). Interestingly, since it has been demonstrated a 10 % variation of T4 levels in normal subjects (Andersen et al. 2002), some authors proposed that CH could be diagnosed in patients with hypothalamic-pituitary diseases followed up for several years showing a 20 % decrease of circulating T4 concentrations of the initial T4 determination (Alexopoulou et al. 2004). From a practical point of view, CH is diagnosed when a patient show low free T4 levels in the presence of reduced or inappropriately normal TSH levels (Lania et al. 2008).

7.4.2   Treatment

Restoration and maintenance of euthyroidism is the therapeutic goal in CH. The majority of patients is actually treated with standard levothyroxine (L-T4) therapy (Lania et al. 2008), the combined treatment with thyroxine plus triiodothyronine not having been proved to be more effective than thyroxine alone in the treatment of all forms of hypothyroidism (Clyde et al. 2003). Before L-T4 therapy is started, a

Table 7.5 L-T4 replacement therapy in children

Age	L-T4 dose (µg/kg/day)
0–3 months	10–15
4–6 months	8–10
1–5 years	5–6
6–12 years	4–5
>12 years/puberty incomplete	2–3
>12 years/puberty complete	1.5–1.7

concomitant condition of central adrenal insufficiency should be excluded to prevent an adrenal crisis unmasked by euthyroidism restoration. If adrenal function cannot be evaluated prior to L-T4 start, it is advisable to begin a prophylactic treatment with steroids (i.e., hydrocortisone or cortone acetate).

Unlike for primary hypothyroidism, serum TSH levels cannot be used in monitoring L-T4 therapy. In fact, several authors demonstrated that low doses of L-T4 are sufficient to completely suppress TSH secretion in the majority of CH patients (Ferretti et al. 1999; Shimon et al. 2002); this finding possibly reflects an abnormal sensitivity in the negative feedback mechanism. In this respect, Shimon et al. suggested that TSH levels above 1.0 mU/l may reflect insufficient replacement (Shimon et al. 2002). In CH, free thyroid hormones should be measured to evaluate the adequacy of L-T4 treatment.

L-thyroxine treatment should be started at low daily dosage and then gradually increased by 25 mcg every 2–3 weeks in order to reach full replacement dose. It has been demonstrated that in the majority of CH patients, normal free T4 and free T3 circulating levels are reached with L-T4 daily dose of 1.5–1.6 mcg/kg BW, these doses being similar to those commonly used in patients with primary hypothyroidism (Lania et al. 2008). In children, the dose is higher that dose used in adults varies according to age (Table 7.5).

When treating CH patients, L-T4 doses depend on the age of CH patients or concomitant treatments. In particular, concomitant estrogens or GH replacement therapies require a significant increase in L-T4 doses to normalize free thyroid hormones levels (Porretti et al. 2002). As far as estrogens are concerned, the increase in L-T4 requirement could be the consequence of the transient increase of thyroxine-binding globulin levels induced by estrogen replacement therapy.

References

Abdu TA, Neary R, Elhadd TA, Akber M et al (2001) Coronary risk in growth hormone deficient hypopituitary adults: increased predicted risk is due largely to lipid profile abnormalities. Clin Endocrinol (Oxf) 55:209–216

Aimaretti G, Corneli G, Razzore P et al (1998) Comparison between insulin-induced hypoglycemia and growth hormone (GH)-releasing hormone + arginine as provocative tests for the diagnosis of GH deficiency in adults. J Clin Endocrinol Metab 83:1615–1618

Alexopoulou O, Beguin C, De Nayer P et al (2004) Clinical and hormonal characteristics of central hypothyroidism at diagnosis and during follow-up in adult patients. Eur J Endocrinol 150:1–8

Andersen S, Pedersen KM, Bruun NH et al (2002) Narrow individual variations in serum T4 and T3 in normal subjects: a clue to understanding of subclinical thyroid disease. J Clin Endocrinol Metab 87:1068–1072

Attanasio AF, Mo D, Erfurth EM et al (2010) Prevalence of metabolic syndrome in adult hypopituitary growth hormone (GH)-deficient patients before and after GH replacement. J Clin Endocrinol Metab 95:74–81

Baloch Z, Carayon P, Conte-Devolx B et al (2003) Laboratory medicine practice guidelines. Laboratory support for the diagnosis and monitoring of thyroid disease. Thyroid 13:3–126

Basaria S (2014) Male hypogonadism. Lancet 383:1250–1263

Bhasin S, Cunningham GR, Hayes FJ et al (2010) Testosterone therapy in men with androgen deficiency syndromes: an Endocrine Society clinical practice guideline. J Clin Endocrinol Metab 95:2536–2559

Biller BM, Samuels MH, Zagar A et al (2002) Sensitivity and specificity of six tests for the diagnosis of adult GH deficiency. J Clin Endocrinol Metab 87:2067–2079

Burman P, Johansson AG, Siegbahn A et al (1997) Growth hormone (GH)-deficient men are more responsive to GH replacement therapy than women. J Clin Endocrinol Metab 82:550–555

Clyde PW, Harari AE, Getka EJ et al (2003) Combined levothyroxine plus liothyronine compared with levothyroxine alone in primary hypothyroidism. A randomized controlled trial. JAMA 290:2952–2958

Corneli G, Di Somma C, Baldelli R et al (2005) The cut-off limits of the GH response to GH-releasing hormone-arginine test related to body mass index. Eur J Endocrinol 153:257–264

Crowley RK, Hamnvik OP, O'Sullivan EP et al (2010) Morbidity and mortality in patients with craniopharyngioma after surgery. Clin Endocrinol (Oxf) 73:516–521

Crowley RK, Argese N, Tomlinson JW et al (2014) Central hypoadrenalism. J Clin Endocrinol Metab 99:4027–4036

Darzy KH, Aimaretti G, Wieringa G et al (2003) The usefulness of the combined growth hormone (GH)-releasing hormone and arginine stimulation test in the diagnosis of radiation-induced GH deficiency is dependent on the post-irradiation time interval. J Clin Endocrinol Metab 88:95–102

Dunkel L, Quinton R (2014) Transition in endocrinology: induction of puberty. Eur J Endocrinol 170:R229–R239

Ferretti E, Persani L, Jaffrain-Rea ML et al (1999) Evaluation of the adequacy of l-T4 replacement therapy in patients with central hypothyroidism. J Clin Endocrinol Metab 84:924–929

Finkelstein JS, Yu EW, Burnett-Bowie SA (2013) Gonadal steroids and body composition, strength, and sexual function in men. N Engl J Med 369:1011–1022

Garnett MR, Puget S, Grill J, Sainte-Rose C (2007) Craniopharyngioma. Orphanet J Rare Dis 10(2):18

Gazzaruso C, Gola M, Karamouzis I et al (2014) Cardiovascular risk in adult patients with growth hormone (GH) deficiency and following substitution with GH-an update. J Clin Endocrinol Metab 99:18–29

Giavoli C, Libé R, Corbetta S et al (2004) Effect of recombinant human growth hormone (GH) replacement on the hypothalamic-pituitary-adrenal axis in adult GH-deficient patients. J Clin Endocrinol Metab 89:5397–5401

Grossman AB (2010) Clinical review#: the diagnosis and management of central hypoadrenalism. J Clin Endocrinol Metab 95:4855–4863

Growth Hormone Research Society (2000) Consensus guidelines for the diagnosis and treatment of growth hormone (GH) deficiency in childhood and adolescence: summary statement of the GH Research Society. GH Research Society. J Clin Endocrinol Metab 85:3988–3989

Hahner S, Allolio B (2009) Therapeutic management of adrenal insufficiency. Best Pract Res Clin Endocrinol Metab 23:167–179

Han TS, Bouloux PM (2010) What is the optimal therapy for young males with hypogonadotropic hypogonadism? Clin Endocrinol (Oxf) 72:731–737

Hartman ML, Crowe BJ, Biller BM et al (2002) Which patients do not require a GH stimulation test for the diagnosis of adult GH deficiency? J Clin Endocrinol Metab 287:477–485

Hayes FJ, Seminara SB, Crowley WF Jr (1998) Hypogonadotropic hypogonadism. Endocrinol Metab Clin North Am 27:739–763

Hoffman AR, Strasburger CJ, Zagar A et al (2004) Efficacy and tolerability of an individualized dosing regimen for adult growth hormone replacement therapy in comparison with fixed body weight-based dosing. J Clin Endocrinol Metab 89:3224–3233

Holmes SJ, Economou G, Whitehouse RW et al (1994) Reduced bone mineral density in patients with adult onset growth hormone deficiency. J Clin Endocrinol Metab 78:669–674

Irwig MS (2013) Male hypogonadism and skeletal health. Curr Opin Endocrinol Diabetes Obes 20:517–522

Johannsson G, Bergthorsdottir R, Nilsson AG et al (2009) Improving glucocorticoid replacement therapy using a novel modified-release hydrocortisone tablet: a pharmacokinetic study. Eur J Endocrinol 161:119–130

Johannsson G, Nilsson AG, Bergthorsdottir R et al (2012) Improved cortisol exposure-time profile and outcome in patients with adrenal insufficiency: a prospective randomized trial of a novel hydrocortisone dual-release formulation. J Clin Endocrinol Metab 97:473–481

Karavitaki N, Brufani C, Warner JT et al (2005) Craniopharyngiomas in children and adults: systematic analysis of 121 cases with long-term follow-up. Clin Endocrinol (Oxf) 62:397–409

Karavitaki N, Cudlip S, Adams CB et al (2006a) Craniopharyngiomas. Endocr Rev 27:371–397

Karavitaki N, Warner JT, Marland A et al (2006b) GH replacement does not increase the risk of recurrence in patients with craniopharyngioma. Clin Endocrinol (Oxf) 64:556–560

Kaufman JM, Taelman P, Vermeulen A et al (1992) Bone mineral status growth hormone-deficient males with isolated and multiple pituitary deficiencies of childhood onset. J Clin Endocrinol Metab 74:118–123

Kazlauskaite R, Evans AT, Villabona CV, Consortium for Evaluation of Corticotropin Test in Hypothalamic-Pituitary Adrenal Insufficiency, et al (2008) Corticotropin tests for hypothalamic-pituitary- adrenal insufficiency: a metaanalysis. J Clin Endocrinol Metab 93:4245–4253

Lania A, Persani L, Beck-Peccoz P (2008) Central hypothyroidism. Pituitary 11:181–186

Lombardi G, Di Somma C, Grasso LF et al (2012) The cardiovascular system in growth hormone excess and growth hormone deficiency. J Endocrinol Invest 35:1021–1029

Misra M (2012) Effects of hypogonadism on bone metabolism in female adolescents and young adults. Nat Rev Endocrinol 8:395–404

Molitch ME, Clemmons DR, Malozowski S et al (2011) Evaluation and treatment of adult growth hormone deficiency: an endocrine society clinical practice guideline. J Clin Endocrinol Metab 96:1587–1609

Moock J, Albrecht C, Friedrich N et al (2009) Health-related quality of life and IGF-1 in GH-deficient adult patients on GH replacement therapy: analysis of the German KIMS data and the Study of Health in Pomerania. Eur J Endocrinol 16:17–24

Müller HL (2014) Craniopharyngioma. Endocr Rev 35:513–543

Øksnes M, Ross R, Løvås K (2015) Optimal glucocorticoid replacement in adrenal insufficiency. Best Pract Res Clin Endocrinol Metab 29:3–15

Porretti S, Giavoli C, Ronchi C et al (2002) Recombinant human GH replacement therapy and thyroid function in a large group of adult GH-deficient patients: when does L-T(4) therapy become mandatory? J Clin Endocrinol Metab 87:2042–2045

Rogol AD (2005) New facets of androgen replacement therapy during childhood and adolescence. Expert Opin Pharmacother 6:1319–1336

Rosner W, Auchus RJ, Azziz R et al (2007) Position statement: utility, limitations, and pitfalls in measuring testosterone: an Endocrine Society position statement. J Clin Endocrinol Metab 92:405–413

Shimon I, Cohen O, Lubetsky A et al (2002) Thyrotropin suppression by thyroid hormone replacement is correlated with thyroxine level normalization in central hypothyroidism. Thyroid 12:823–827

Silveira LF, Latronico AC (2013) Approach to the patient with hypogonadotropic hypogonadism. J Clin Endocrinol Metab 98:1781–1788

Smith MR, Finkelstein JS, McGovern FJ et al (2002) Changes in body composition during androgen deprivation therapy for prostate cancer. J Clin Endocrinol Metab 87:599–603

Wüster C, Abs R, Bengtsson BA et al (2001) The influence of growth hormone deficiency, growth hormone replacement therapy and other aspects of hypopituitarism on fracture rate and bone mineral density. J Bone Miner Res 2:398–405

Zitzmann M, Nieschlag E (2000) Hormone substitution in male hypogonadism. Mol Cell Endocrinol 161:73–88

Metabolic Consequences: Obesity and Energy Expenditure, Can They Be Treated?

Valentina Lo Preiato, Valentina Vicennati, Renato Pasquali, and Uberto Pagotto

Abstract

Obesity and hypopituitarism are major side effects of craniopharyngiomas. Awareness of the presence of obesity and/or food-seeking behavior in patients affected by acquired pathologic processes damaging the hypothalamic centers is highly recommended. The craniopharyngiomas cause structural damage to the hypothalamus before or, more often, after surgery. These tumors may occur at any age but are more common in childhood and adolescence. Obesity may often appear before any therapeutic approach is attempted. Obesity and hyperphagia as a consequence of surgical or radiotherapy treatment must be managed with particular care.

This chapter will try to highlight the potential medical and surgical treatments to limit obesity, hyperphagia, and alterations in energy expenditure often described in patients affected by craniopharyngioma, elucidating at the same time the mechanisms by which all these metabolic alterations may occur.

V. Lo Preiato • V. Vicennati • R. Pasquali
Division of Endocrinology, Department of Medical and Surgical Science, Centre for Applied Biomedical Research (C.R.B.A.), S. Orsola-Malpighi Hospital, University of Bologna, Bologna, Italy

U. Pagotto (✉)
Division of Endocrinology, Department of Medical and Surgical Science, Centre for Applied Biomedical Research (C.R.B.A.), S. Orsola-Malpighi Hospital, University of Bologna, Bologna, Italy

Division of Endocrinology, Centre for Applied Biomedical Research (C.R.B.A.), S. Orsola-Malpighi Hospital, Bologna, Italy
e-mail: uberto.pagotto@unibo.it

© Springer International Publishing Switzerland 2016
A. Lania et al. (eds.), *Diagnosis and Management of Craniopharyngiomas: Key Current Topics*, DOI 10.1007/978-3-319-22297-4_8

8.1   Introduction

Obesity and hypopituitarism are major side effects of childhood and adolescent craniopharyngioma (CP). In the case of hypopituitarism, replacement therapy must be started immediately. However, weight gain occurs despite adequate endocrine hormone replacement therapy being established (Muller 2014). At the diagnosis of craniopharyngioma, less than 20 % of patients are obese, but after surgery, the percentage increases over 50 % (Poretti et al. 2004; Page-Wilson et al. 2012; Muller 2014). After surgical treatment, most of the weight gain frequently occurs during the first year (Muller et al. 2001; Holmer et al. 2010). The major risk factor for development of obesity in craniopharyngioma is the involvement of the hypothalamic area, by tumor or surgical/irradiation damage (Muller et al. 2001; Müller et al. 2004). In fact, some studies show that in tumors that do not involved the mammillary bodies, sparing surgery and the experience of the surgeon decreases the risk of obesity occurence (Müller et al. 2011a; Elowe-Grau et al. 2013). Patients with hypothalamic damage have disorders of circadian rhythms, appetite, energy balance, and autonomic nervous system equilibrium. These alterations promote obesity onset and make any type of therapeutic approach for this problem poorly effective (Muller 2014). Nevertheless, weight control is very important for the prognosis of craniopharyngioma because weight gain usually causes a substantial decrease in quality of life and an increased risk of sleep apnea syndrome, metabolic syndrome, cardiovascular disease, and sudden death events (Muller et al. 2001; Muller 2014).

8.2   Lifestyle Therapy

Given the high percentage of patients who develop hypothalamic obesity (HO), it is essential to prevent the weight increase right from the diagnosis of CP (Rakhshani et al. 2010). The first approach for the treatment of HO is a scrupulous nutritional assessment, because up to 25 % of patients are hyperphagic. Although the mechanisms involved in the development of hyperphagia are not yet fully known, many studies show that the dysregulation of hunger may occur at many levels (Page-Wilson et al. 2012). A recent study used functional magnetic resonance imaging to show that patients with CP have an altered satiety perception. The activity of some cerebral areas (bilateral nucleus accumbens, insula and medial orbitofrontal cortex) was evaluated before and after a meal in four CP patients versus age- and weight-matched controls. After the meal, the controls showed less activation of these specific brain areas by visual food cues, while CP subjects did not show this kind of adaptive response, disclosing that the perception of food stimuli is altered in HO (Roth et al. 2012). In addition, numerous studies show altered levels of hormones involved in the sense of hunger regulation. Roth et al. compared the ghrelin and insulin levels, homeostasis model assessment of insulin resistance (HOMA), and quantitative insulin sensitivity check index (QUICKI) in normal-weight and obese subjects with CP versus BMI-, gender-, and age-matched controls. Obese CP patients had significantly higher baseline and postmeal insulin, higher HOMA, and lower QUICKI and ghrelin (probably secondary to hyperinsulinemia) (Roth et al. 2011). Another study demonstrated that the decrease of ghrelin levels after glucose load is significantly smaller in CP than in nonfunctioning pituitary adenoma patients (NFPA). In fact, nonfunctioning pituitary adenomas do not typically affect the diencephalic area. This study also showed that basal and 60-min-after-glucose-intake leptin levels were significantly higher in CP subjects compared with NFPA. This suggests the existence of leptin resistance in CP that contributes to the onset of hyperphagia and obesity in these patients (Roth et al. 1998; Roemmler-Zehrer et al. 2014). When food-seeking is present, strongly behavioral supervision is obviously the first approach for management of HO and is absolutely necessary to prevent massive weight gain.

Even if food intake is normal, CP subjects show a reduction of physical activity that contributes to explain the obesity onset. This decrease is determined by numerous factors. Some patients present neurological and visual deficits that may cause a restricted range of movements. Furthermore, CP patients show a disturbed melatonin secretion resulting in increased daytime sleepiness (Müller et al. 2002). Finally, replacement therapy of hypothalamic-pituitary-adrenal axis cannot faithfully replicate the physiological changes. At some times during the day, patients may thus be undertreated and feel more tired (Harz et al. 2003). Despite all these limiting factors, physical activity should always be encouraged to increase energy expenditure.

In addition to this, another major problem of HO resides in a disturbed energy homeostasis. Numerous studies have shown the presence of hyperactivation of the vagal system and a deficiency of the sympathetic system that determine a dysregulation of energy balance (Holmer et al. 2010; Kim et al. 2010). The disinhibited parasympathetic activity caused by ventromedial hypothalamic damage induces postmeal insulin hypersecretion from pancreatic beta cells, resulting in increased energy storage (Muller 2014; Lustig et al. 2003; Lustig 2011; Cohen et al. 2013). On the other hand, a reduced activation of the sympathetic nervous system has been repeatedly found in HO (Schöfl et al. 2002; Roth et al. 2007; Cohen et al. 2013). Roth et al. showed that patients with CP had lower urine homovanillic acid (HVA) and urine vanillylmandelic acid (VMA), markers of catecholamine turnover (Roth et al. 2007). Besides, the induction of hypoglycemia determines a significantly lower increase of epinephrine in CP patients compared to controls (Coutant et al. 2003). All these values suggest decreased sympathetic activity, contributing to cause massive obesity. The presence of these orthosympathetic and parasympathetic system alterations causes significant difficulties in the management of HO and explains the lack of effectiveness of the lifestyle approach in these patients.

In conclusion, low caloric diet and increased physical activity must absolutely be the first-line therapy for obesity, also in craniopharyngioma. However, even if the patients change their lifestyle appropriately, the results on weight are lower compared to healthy subjects and may often be inadequate and disappointing.

8.3   Pharmacotherapy

Considering the specific mechanisms involved in the genesis of HO, some studies have been conducted to test drugs that could increase orthosympathetic activity and possibly energy expenditure (Table 8.1).

Table 8.1 Results of different drugs used in obesity craniopharyngioma

Article	Drugs	Number of patients (patients with CP)	Results	Period of treatment	Adverse effects
Mason et al. (2002)	Dextroamphetamine	5 (5)	Mean of BMI was modified from 32 ± 2.8 (initial) to 31 ± 3.3 (after treatment)	24 months	One child complained of headaches with 5 mg daily, regressed with 2.5 mg daily
Ismail et al. (2006)	Dextroamphetamine	12 (9)	-0.7 BMI-SDS in males, -0.44 BMI-SDS in females	15 months	One patient complained of insomnia
Elfers and Roth (2011)	Methylphenidate	1 (1)	BMI decreased from 45.5 to 41.4 kg/m^2	87 weeks	No data
Danielsson et al. (2007)	Sibutramine	50 (4)	Mean -0.8 BMI-SDS respect initial BMI-SDS	6 weeks	No data
Lustig et al. (1999)	Octreotide	8	Mean weight loss was -4.8 ± 1.8 kg	6 months	No data
Lustig et al. (2003)	Octreotide	18 (13)	BMI decreased (-0.2 ± 0.2) but weight increased ($+1.6 \pm 0.6$)	6 months	Four subjects exhibited gallstone, abdominal discomfort, and diarrhea which resolved in the 2nd month of therapy. Two subjects developed mild glucose intolerance
	Octreotide	60	Nonchanging BMI	6 months	Terminated earlier for increased risk of gallstone
Hamilton et al. (2011)	Diazoxide + metformin	9 (9)	Mean BMI and BMI-SDS decreased (respectively -0.3 ± 2.3 and -0.04 ± 0.15)	6 months	
Müller et al. (2006)	Melatonin	10 (10)	Morning and nighttime melatonin levels were related to BMI. Administration of melatonin improved sleepiness, but it has an unclear effect on BMI.		Vomiting and peripheral edema that caused the withdrawal of two patients

Article	Drugs	Number of patients (patients with CP)	Results	Period of treatment	Adverse effects
Zoicas et al. (2013)	GLP1 analogue	9 (6)	Weight loss was −13.1 ± 5.1 kg (−9 to −22 kg)	51 months	Nausea and vomiting that caused the withdrawal of one patient
Greenway and Bray (2008)	Caffeine+ephedrine	3 (2)	Patient 1 (CP): −9 % of initial body weight in 3 months. Weight was stabilized for 2 years Patient 2 (CP): lost 18.8 % of initial body weight in 6 months. Six years after, the weight loss was −9.5 % compared to the beginning. Patient 3: lost 14 % of initial body weight in 6 months, but after this time, the weight loss was arrested and returned to the initial weight after 5 years		No adverse effect has been reported
Article	Drugs	Number of patients (patients with CP)	Results	Period of treatment	Adverse effects
	Beloranib	14	Mean weight loss: −3.4 kg	4 weeks	No serious adverse effects reported
	Orlistat	No data in HO			
	Phentermine	No data in HO			Constipation, xerostomia, insomnia, and fluctuation in mood

(continued)

Table 8.1 (continued)

A summary of obesity craniopharyngioma bariatric therapy

Article	Type of bariatric surgery	Number of patients	Results
Müller et al. (2007)	LAGB	4	Patient 1: from +13.9 BMI-SDS to +9.9 BMI-SDS in 4 years Patient 2: from +10.3 BMI-SDS to +9.7 BMI-SDS in 1.5 years Patient 3: from +11.4 BMI-SDS to +9.5 BMI-SDS in 3 years Patient 4: from +7.3 BMI-SDS to +5.9 BMI-SDS in 2.5 years
Inge et al. (2007)	RYGB	1	Lost 49 kg in 2.5 years
Schultes et al. (2009)	Distal gastric bypass surgery	1	Lost 54 kg in 1 year
Bretault et al. (2013)	6 LAGB 8 SG 6 RYGB 1 BPD	21	At 6 months: RYGB: −18.6 % of initial weight SG: −20.7 % of initial weight LAGB: −10.5 % of initial weight BPD: −11.3 % of initial weight At 12 months: RYGB: −20.2 % of initial weight SG: −19.6 % of initial weight LAGB: −6.1 % of initial weight BPD: −24.8 % of initial weight

Mason et al. used dextroamphetamine (a potent central nervous system stimulant by inhibiting the reuptake of dopamine, norepinephrine, and serotonin) to decrease the weight in five children who had undergone surgical resection for CP and had significant postoperative weight gain. In the 6 months of treatment, BMI stabilized regardless of caloric intake and values before and after were comparable. Patients also appeared less hyperphagic and more active; hence, the resistance to physical exercise was improved (Mason et al. 2002). Similar results were obtained in another study in which 12 children with HO (including 9 with CP) were treated with the same agent (Ismail et al. 2006). Other sympathomimetic drugs producing peripheral adrenergic stimulation to reduce food intake and to increase metabolic rate, such as caffeine and ephedrine, were used in three cases affected by HO (2 had CP). The combination of these two drugs showed that it was possible to lose from 8 to 19 % of weight. Two patients (both with CP) maintained the weight loss for 2 and 6 years, while the third subject regained weight after 6 months, returning to the initial weight after 5 years (Greenway and Bray 2008).

Another central psychomotor stimulant, methylphenidate, used in the treatment of attention deficit hyperactivity disorder (ADHD), was tested in only one patient with HO due to CP. This drug produces an increase in brain synaptic dopamine signaling, determining anorexia. In fact, in this patient, weight gain ceased following the start of methylphenidate treatment and, after 87 weeks, BMI was markedly decreased (from 45.5 to 41.4 kg/m^2) (Elfers and Roth 2011).

Sibutramine has also been used for HO treatment. This drug is an inhibitor of serotonin, norepinephrine, and dopamine reuptake, thereby increasing the levels of these neurotransmitters in synaptic clefts, helping enhance satiety. Sibutramine was tested in patient cohorts with different obesity syndromes (patients with hypothalamic damage; Laurence-Moon-Bardet-Biedl, Prader-Willi, and Down syndromes; mutation in the melanocortin receptor 4; myelomeningocele; mental retardation; autism spectrum disorder; and ADHD). A double-blind, placebo-controlled, crossover trial (20+20 weeks), followed by a 6-month open phase, was performed. During the sibutramine treatment period, BMI, total body fat percentage, and triglyceride plasma levels were significantly lower than in the placebo group. Also in the open phase (in which all subjects were treated with sibutramine), a reduction in weight was observed. Weight results obtained by children with HO were compared to children with non-hypothalamic obesity. The effect of sibutramine was lower in HO, indicating a partial resistance to this drug (Danielsson et al. 2007). However, sibutramine has been withdrawn from the market due to the increased risk of cardiovascular events shown by the Sibutramine Cardiovascular Outcomes (SCOUT) trial.

Phentermine (norepinephrine hypothalamic release stimulator) was recently approved by the FDA (not by the EMA) for the short-term treatment of obesity, as monotherapy or in combination with topiramate, but no data are available in HO (Page-Wilson et al. 2012).

The somatostatin analogue octreotide has also been investigated for HO to limit the hyperinsulinism produced by parasympathetic disinhibition. In an open study of eight patients with HO, 6 months of subcutaneous octreotide achieved significant weight loss, decreasing BMI and reducing insulin secretion in response to oral glucose stimuli in comparison to a 6-month pre-study observation period (Lustig et al. 1999). In another study on 18 patients, the result on hyperinsulinemia was confirmed. While weight loss was not observed, octreotide significantly attenuated weight gain compared to placebo. In addition, improvement in spontaneous physical activity was noted with octreotide (Lustig et al. 2003). These studies were followed by a larger trial using octreotide in 60 patients with HO. After 6 months, it showed no efficacy in changing BMI, and the open-label segment of this study was terminated earlier than planned due to an increased risk of gallstones (http://clinicaltrials.gov/ct2/show/NCT0076362). Diazoxide (a potassium channel activator, which inhibits insulin secretion) mixed with metformin was recently used in nine obese subjects treated for CP for 6 months, after at least 6 months of lifestyle therapy. In patients completing the study (seven of nine), weight gain during the study was significantly reduced compared to the 6-month pre-study, and three subjects reduced their weight during the treatment (Hamilton et al. 2011).

Melatonin regulation is also altered in CP patients. A lack of melatonin may contribute to the occurrence of daytime sleepiness and decreased spontaneous physical activity typically observed in these subjects. Hence, melatonin replacement has also been studied in HO. In a study on ten subjects with CP and daytime sleepiness, supplements of melatonin determined an improvement of daytime somnolence and spontaneous physical activity, although it did not clearly impact on BMI (Müller et al. 2006).

Another approach to HO management is the use of GLP1 analogues, recently approved by the FDA and EMA for the treatment of obesity. In a recent study, nine patients with HO (six with CP) were treated with exenatide (eight) or liraglutide (last one). Significant weight loss was achieved in all subjects completing the study (one patient treated with exenatide reported unendurable nausea and vomiting and therefore left the study). Improved insulin resistance (HOMA-IR) and glycate hemoglobin values were reported (Zoicas et al. 2013). Based on these positive results, a larger study was started (still in progress) on patients with genetic hypothalamic obesity.

Moreover, enrollment in a Phase 2a clinical trial (ZAF-221) testing beloranib for the treatment of HO was completed at the start of 2015. This drug is a novel injectable small molecule which inhibits methionine aminopeptidase 2 (MetAP2), an enzyme that modulates the activity of key cellular processes that control metabolism. MetAP2 inhibitors reduce the tone of signals that drive lipid synthesis by the liver and fat storage. MetAP2 inhibition thus increases metabolism of fat and induces weight loss and hunger reduction (Fig. 8.1). The ZAF-221 trial is a randomized, double-blind, placebo-controlled trial in which patients will receive twice-weekly subcutaneous injections of 1.8 mg beloranib or placebo. This trial enrolled 14 obese patients (nine women and five men) who were confirmed by magnetic resonance imaging (MRI) to have had hypothalamic injury. The primary outcome measure is change in body weight. Secondary outcomes include changes in the patient's lipid profile, CRP (C-reactive protein, a marker of systemic inflammation), sense of hunger, and quality of life. After 4 weeks of treatment, beloranib treatment resulted in a

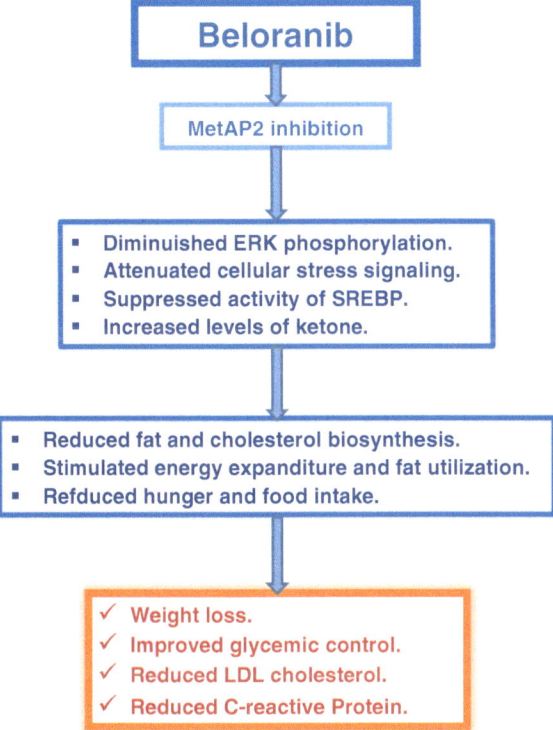

Fig. 8.1 Mechanism of action of beloranib. Beloranib is an inhibitor of methionine aminopeptidases (MetAP2). MetAPs are enzymes responsible for the removal of methionine from the amino-terminus of newly synthesized proteins, crucial passage for amino terminal modifications (acetylation and myristoylation of glycine) and for protein stability. The precise mechanism for the anti-obesity effect of MetAP2 inhibitors is not well known. However, probably MetAP2 inhibition results into suppression of the activity of sterol regulatory element binding protein (SREBP), reducing lipid and cholesterol biosynthesis via ERK-related pathways. MetAP2 inhibition also reduces the factors involved in inflammation and increases the levels of adiponectin. Beloranib seems to increase levels of ketone bodies (beta-hydroxybutyrate), suggesting that MetAP2 inhibition stimulates energy expenditure, fat utilization, and lipid excretion

mean weight loss of 3.4 kg in contrast to 0.3 kg mean weight loss in placebo-treated patients ($p=0.01$). Improvements in cardiovascular disease risk factors of lipids and inflammation (measured by CRP) were also observed. However recently, it was learned of a patient with Prader Willi Syndrome death occurred in randomized, double-blind phase, placebo-controlled trial. The cause of death remains unknown at this time, but, as required by standard practice, the event was reported to the Food and Drug Administration and it is under investigation for the understanding this event (http://ir.zafgen.com/releasedetail.cfm?ReleaseID=936610).

Finally, orlistat, an inhibitor of pancreatic and gastrointestinal lipases that blocks dietary fat absorption, is approved for weight loss, but has not been formally studied in patients with HO. However, its use may be considered in clinical practice (Page-Wilson et al. 2012).

In conclusion, many pharmacological weapons have been used to tackle obesity, but the poor results make new research vital to find more effective drugs in the future.

8.4 Surgery

Bariatric surgery has shown excellent results in terms of weight loss, ameliorating morbidity, and reducing mortality in obese subjects. However, the specific mechanisms underlying the development of HO (in particular, dysregulation of appetite that makes compliance with postoperative dietary restrictions difficult) mean that the bariatric approach has been used only in a few cases. Despite the limited data in the literature, bariatric surgery seems to show encouraging results, at least in the short term.

Muller et al. performed laparoscopic adjustable gastric banding (LAGB) in four children with craniopharyngioma who had shown a serious weight increase after surgery for tumor. After follow-up lasting from 2.5 to 4.5 years, BMI decreased continuously in all patients. Eating behavior improved considerably; in particular, addiction to sweet things was reduced significantly. Of the four subjects, in two the LAGB became dislocated, causing a temporary recovery of the weight; however, after the repositioning reoperation, the weight loss continued (Müller et al. 2007). The continuing follow-up of these patients (5–9 years after LAGB) showed that all patients recovered weight gradually but remained at a level comparable to the level at the time of LABG. Only one subject, poorly compliant, exceeded the pre-LAGB weight, from a BMI of 51.9 at the time of LAGB to 53.6 at the last examination (5 years later) (Müller et al. 2011b). LAGB is the most acceptable surgical choice due to its reversibility, a positive factor in the pediatric population. However, other approaches have been proposed for HO, such as Roux-en-Y gastric bypass (RYGB). After CP surgery, a 14-year-old child developed hyperphagia, weight gain (70 kg/year), significant hyperinsulinism, left ventricular hypertrophy, and obstructive sleep apnea syndrome (despite diet, demanding physical activity and octreotide treatment) and thus underwent RYGB with anterior truncal vagotomy at the age of 18 years. After the bariatric approach, the hyperphagia, food craving, and weight decreased (−49 kg), and hypertrophy was resolved. Fasting insulin was normalized by 14 months (Inge et al. 2007; Bingham et al. 2012). Similar results were obtained with distal gastric bypass surgery in a 29-year-old man who had undergone craniopharyngioma resection at age 8: 18 months after the bariatric operation, BMI had decreased, hunger was markedly ameliorated, and type II diabetes was in remission (Schultes et al. 2009). A systematic review of 21 bariatric operations in CP patients (six LAGB, eight sleeve gastrectomies, six RYGB, and one biliopancreatic diversion) was performed. At 6 months, the mean weight loss was greater in the RYGB group (−31 kg) than sleeve gastrectomy (−28.3 kg) or LAGB (−12.9 kg). The same results were observed at 12 months (−33.7 kg versus −25.9 kg and −7.5 kg, respectively). Weight change was maximal at 6 months for LAGB and sleeve gastrectomy (SG), while it was highest at 12 months for RYGB. Nevertheless, restrictive procedures may be safer due to the shorter hospitalization and the lower risk for mineral and vitamin deficit (Bretault et al. 2013). Finally, to reduce the vagal hyperactivation and insulin hypersecretion often observed in HO patients, vagotomy has been proposed as another surgical approach. This operation has provided opposing results – positive (Smith et al. 1983) and failures (Fobi 1993) – and was thus abandoned for many years. However, it has recently been resumed without pyloromyotomy, and preliminary data suggest promising results (Lustig et al. 2009).

Concluding, although bariatric surgery seems to show encouraging results, it should only be used as a last treatment and only in complicated cases. This approach requires a highly experienced surgical team and a careful follow-up. Furthermore, the data now available are very few, and it is absolutely necessary to expand them through randomized trials.

Conclusions

Craniopharyngioma is a histologically benign tumor, but it often requires extensive surgery involving the peri-diencephalic area, determining panhypopituitarism and obesity. This increase in weight is a very serious problem because it is conspicuous, has a fast onset, and is difficult to stop. In a few months, the massive fat increase determines the rapid onset of many problems such as hyperlipidemia, hypertriglyceridemia, severe steatosis, diabetes, hypertension, cardiovascular problems, OSAS, and skeletal problems. Hypothalamic obesity is supported by highly complex mechanisms. In particular, the hyperphagia and reduced energy expenditure by the tissues are very difficult to fight. For this reason, the lifestyle approach and the currently available drugs achieve disappointing results. Since CP affects pediatric subjects, bariatric surgery and especially the definitive approaches have long been avoided because they are considered too dangerous. However, the few data available on bariatric surgery seem to show its effectiveness, at least in the short term. Nevertheless, it is necessary to confirm the initial results obtained with randomized trials.

References

Bingham NC, Rose SR, Inge TH (2012) Bariatric surgery in hypothalamic obesity. Front Endocrinol (Lausanne) 14:3–23

Bretault M, Boillot A, Muzard L et al (2013) Clinical review: bariatric surgery following treatment for craniopharyngioma: a systematic review and individual-level data meta-analysis. J Clin Endocrinol Metab 98(6):2239–2246

Cohen M, Syme C, McCrindle BW et al (2013) Autonomic nervous system balance in children and adolescents with craniopharyngioma and hypothalamic obesity. Eur J Endocrinol 168(6):845–852

Coutant R, Maurey H, Rouleau S et al (2003) Defect in epinephrine production in children with craniopharyngioma: functional or organic origin? J Clin Endocrinol Metab 88(12):5969–5975

Danielsson P, Janson A, Norgren S et al (2007) Impact sibutramine therapy in children with hypothalamic obesity or obesity with aggravating syndromes. J Clin Endocrinol Metab 92(11):4101–4106

Elfers CT, Roth CL (2011) Effects of methylphenidate on weight gain and food intake in hypothalamic obesity. Front Endocrinol (Lausanne) 2:78

Elowe-Gruau E, Beltrand J, Brauner R et al (2013) Childhood craniopharyngioma: hypothalamus-sparing surgery decreases the risk of obesity. J Clin Endocrinol Metab 98(6):2376–2382

Fobi MA (1993) Operations that are questionable for the control of obesity. Obes Surg 3:197–200

Greenway FL, Bray GA (2008) Treatment of hypothalamic obesity with caffeine and ephedrine. Endocr Pract 14(6):697–703

Hamilton JK, Conwell LS, Syme C et al (2011) Hypothalamic obesity following craniopharyngioma surgery: results of a pilot trial of combined Diazoxide and metformin therapy. Int J Pediatr Endocrinol 2011:417949

Harz KJ, Müller HL, Waldeck E et al (2003) Obesity in patients with craniopharyngioma: assessment of food intake and movement counts indicating physical activity. J Clin Endocrinol Metab 88(11):5227–5231

Holmer H, Pozarek G, Wirfalt E et al (2010) Reduced energy expenditure and impaired feeding-related signals but not high energy intake reinforces hypothalamic obesity in adults with childhood onset craniopharyngioma. J Clin Endocrinol Metab 95(12):5395–5402

Inge TH, Pfluger P, Zeller M et al (2007) Gastric bypass surgery for treatment of hypothalamic obesity after craniopharyngioma therapy. Nat Clin Pract Endocrinol Metab 3(8):606–609

Ismail D, O'Connell MA, Zacharin MR (2006) Dexamphetamine use for management of obesity and hypersomnolence following hypothalamic injury. J Pediatr Endocrinol Metab 19(2):129–134

Kim RJ, Shah R, Tershakovec AM et al (2010) Energy expenditure in obesity associated with craniopharyngioma. Childs Nerv Syst 26(7):913–917

Lustig RH, Rose SR, Burghen GA et al (1999) Hypothalamic obesity caused by cranial insult in children: altered glucose and insulin dynamics and reversal by a somatostatin agonist. J Pediatr 135(2 Pt 1):162–168

Lustig RH, Hinds PS, Ringwald-Smith K et al (2003) Octreotide therapy of pediatric hypothalamic obesity: a double-blind, placebo-controlled trial. J Clin Endocrinol Metab 88(6):2586–2592

Lustig RH, Tsai P, Hirose S et al (2009) Treatment of hypothalamic obesity by laparoscopic truncal vagotomy: early experience. In: Proceedings of the 8th Lason Wilkins/European Pediatric Endocrine Society Meeting, New York

Lustig RH (2011) Hypothalamic obesity after craniopharyngioma: mechanisms, diagnosis, and treatment. Front Endocrinol (Lausanne) 2:60

Mason PW, Krawiecki N, Meacham LR (2002) The use of dextroamphetamine to treat obesity and hyperphagia in children treated for craniopharyngioma. Arch Pediatr Adolesc Med 156(9):887–892

Muller HL, Bueb K, Barteles U et al (2001) Obesity after childhood craniopharyngioma – German multicenter study on pre-operative risk factors and quality of life. Klin Pediatr 213:244–249

Müller HL, Handwerker G, Wollny B et al (2002) Melatonin secretion and increased daytime sleepiness in childhood craniopharyngioma patients. J Clin Endocrinol Metab 87(8):3993–3996

Müller HL, Emser A, Faldum A et al (2004) Longitudinal study on growth and body mass index before and after diagnosis of childhood craniopharyngioma. J Clin Endocrinol Metab 89(7):3298–3305

Müller HL, Handwerker G, Gebhardt U et al (2006) Melatonin treatment in obese patients with childhood craniopharyngioma and increased daytime sleepiness. Cancer Causes Control 17(4):583–589

Müller HL, Gebhardt U, Wessel V et al (2007) First experiences with laparoscopic adjustable gastric banding (LAGB) in the treatment of patients with childhood craniopharyngioma and morbid obesity. Klin Padiatr 219(6):323–325

Müller HL, Gebhardt U, Maroske J et al (2011a) Long-term follow-up of morbidly obese patients with childhood craniopharyngioma after laparoscopic adjustable gastric banding (LAGB). Klin Padiatr 223:372–373

Müller HL, Gebhardt U, Teske C et al (2011b) Post-operative hypothalamic lesions and obesity in childhood craniopharyngioma: results of the multinational prospective trial KRANIOPHARYNGEOM 2000 after 3-year follow-up. Eur J Endocrinol 165(1):17–24

Muller HL (2014) Craniopharyngioma. Endocr Rev 35(3):513–543

Page-Wilson G, Wardlaw SL, Khandji AG et al (2012) Hypothalamic obesity in patients with craniopharyngioma: treatment approaches and the emerging role of gastric bypass surgery. Pituitary 15(1):84–92

Poretti A, Grotzer MA, Ribi K et al (2004) Outcome of craniopharyngioma in children: long-term complications and quality of life. Dev Med Child Neurol 46:220–229

Rakhshani N, Jeffery AS, Schulte F et al (2010) Evaluation of a comprehensive care clinic model for children with brain tumor and risk for hypothalamic obesity. Obesity (Silver Spring) 18(9):1768–1774

Roemmler-Zehrer J, Geigenberger V, Störmann S et al (2014) Food intake regulating hormones in adult craniopharyngioma patients. Eur J Endocrinol 170(4):627–635

Roth C, Wilken B, Hanefeld F et al (1998) Hyperphagia in children with craniopharyngioma is associated with hyperleptinaemia and a failure in the downregulation of appetite. Eur J Endocrinol 138(1):89–91

Roth CL, Hunneman DH, Gebhardt U et al (2007) Reduced sympathetic metabolites in urine of obese patients with craniopharyngioma. Pediatr Res 61(4):496–501

Roth CL, Gebhardt U, Müller HL (2011) Appetite-regulating hormone changes in patients with craniopharyngioma. Obesity (Silver Spring) 19(1):36–42

Roth CL, Aylward E, Liang O et al (2012) Functional neuroimaging in craniopharyngioma: a useful tool to better understand hypothalamic obesity? Obes Facts 5(2):243–253

Schöfl C, Schleth A, Berger D et al (2002) Sympathoadrenal counterregulation in patients with hypothalamic craniopharyngioma. J Clin Endocrinol Metab 87(2):624–629

Schultes B, Ernst B, Schmid F et al (2009) Distal gastric bypass surgery for the treatment of hypothalamic obesity after childhood craniopharyngioma. Eur J Endocrinol 161(1):201–206

Smith DK, Sarfeh J, Hoard L (1983) Truncal vagotomy in hypothalamic obesity. Lancet 1(8337):1330–1331

Zoicas F, Droste M, Mayr B et al (2013) GLP-1 analogues as a new treatment option for hypothalamic obesity in adults: report of nine cases. Eur J Endocrinol 168(5):699–706

Metabolic Consequences: Electrolyte Disturbances

9

Alessandro Peri

Abstract

Water-electrolyte imbalance may occur in patients with craniopharyngioma. In many cases, this condition is related to an altered pattern of synthesis/secretion of arginine vasopressin, although other factors may contribute to its onset. Arginine vasopressin deficiency, which causes diabetes insipidus, is present at the time of diagnosis of craniopharyngioma in about 15 % of cases and may represent the presenting clinical manifestation of the tumor. The onset of diabetes insipidus may also occur after surgical treatment, more frequently as a consequence of a transcranial approach and very rarely as a consequence of radiotherapy. Postoperative diabetes insipidus appears to be more frequently observed in children than in adults, in males, and in the presence of large intrasellar lesions and cerebrospinal fluid leak. Postoperative diabetes insipidus may be transient, permanent, or triphasic. Triphasic diabetes insipidus is characterized by a first phase of polyuria, followed by a second phase of antidiuresis due to an uncontrolled release of arginine vasopressin. The third phase is characterized by the depletion of arginine vasopressin stores and consequently by permanent diabetes insipidus. Other conditions, such as fluid overload or hypocortisolism, may contribute to the onset of water-electrolyte alterations in patients with craniopharyngioma subjected to surgery. The presence of water-electrolyte alterations and their etiology should be carefully investigated in patients with craniopharyngioma, especially in the perioperative period, in order to promptly initiate the most appropriate treatment and avoid possibly severe consequences.

A. Peri
Department of Experimental and Clinical Biomedical Sciences "Mario Serio", Endocrine Unit, "Center for Research, Transfer and High Education on Chronic, Inflammatory, Degenerative and Neoplastic Disorders for the Development of Novel Therapies" (DENOThe), University of Florence, Florence, Italy
e-mail: alessandro.peri@unifi.it

© Springer International Publishing Switzerland 2016
A. Lania et al. (eds.), *Diagnosis and Management of Craniopharyngiomas: Key Current Topics*, DOI 10.1007/978-3-319-22297-4_9

9.1 Introduction

Water-electrolyte disturbances may be encountered in patients with craniopharyngioma (CP). This is not surprising, if we consider the anatomical proximity of this type of lesion to the hypothalamus, pituitary, optic chiasm, and internal carotid artery. The main culprit for water-electrolyte imbalance in CP appears to be arginine vasopressin (AVP), which is synthesized in the supraoptic and paraventricular nuclei of the hypothalamus and released by the axon terminals of the neurohypophysis. However, other factors that will be discussed in this chapter may be involved in the etiopathogenesis of this condition.

9.2 CP and Presurgical Electrolyte Alterations

AVP deficiency, which causes diabetes insipidus (DI), may be present at the time of diagnosis of CP. Acquired central DI appears to occur preoperatively in about 15 % of cases (ranging from 6 to 38 %), both in children and in adults, according to clinical series (Pratheesh et al. 2013; Müller et al. 2003; Karavitaki et al. 2005; Karavitaki and Wass 2008; Müller 2010). In 15 % of patients, DI appears as the presenting clinical manifestation that requires the attention of a physician (Karavitaki et al. 2005). Particular attention requires a DI of sudden onset, because it may suggest the presence of a tumoral proliferation, mostly a craniopharyngioma or a germinoma if it occurs before the age of 30 years, whereas after the age of 50 years a brain metastasis should be considered first (Leroy et al. 2013).

9.3 Postsurgical Electrolyte Alterations

At variance with other endocrine alterations, which do not appear to be influenced by the type of treatment, DI is probably more common in surgically treated patients (Karavitaki et al. 2005; Karavitaki et al. 2006). The resection of certain types of lesions, including CP, Rathke-cleft cysts, and ACTH-secreting adenomas, appears more frequently associated with DI (Hensen et al. 1999; Nemergut et al. 2005). In patients with CP, it is reported to occur with a variable frequency after surgery, ranging from 25 to 86 % of cases (Karavitaki et al. 2006), and appears to be more frequently observed in children than in adults, according to the series of patients reported by Pratesh et al. (80 % vs. 63 %) (Pratheesh et al. 2013). Besides young age, other factors that likely increase the risk of postsurgical DI include male sex, large intrasellar lesions, and cerebrospinal fluid leak (Hensen et al. 1999; Nemergut et al. 2005). There is evidence that there is no reversal of a preexisting AVP deficiency, and therefore, if DI is already present at the time of diagnosis, it is expected to be present also after surgical removal of the tumor (Karavitaki et al. 2005). The same occurs for anterior pituitary hormone deficiencies, which very often persist after surgery in CP (Thomsett et al. 1980; Hetelekidis et al. 1993; Paja et al. 1995; Honegger et al. 1999), whereas restoration of preexisting hormone deficiencies after surgery is more likely to occur in the case of pituitary adenomas (Ahmed et al. 1999; Murad et al. 2010).

The type of surgical approach may have a role on the new onset of DI. For the transcranial approach, the rate of newly diagnosed DI ranges from 43 to 79 % of patients, whereas in endonasal series, 8–48 % of patients developed DI (Fatemi et al. 2009; Fahlbusch et al. 1999; Van Effenterre and Boch 2002; Karavitaki et al. 2005; Cavallo et al. 2009; Gardner et al. 2008; Jane et al. 2010; Campbell et al. 2010). The improved visualization of the infundibulum, pituitary stalk, and superior hypophyseal branches probably explains these differences.

The presence of DI after surgery appears to have also a prognostic role, because it has been suggested that the metabolic consequences of AVP deficiency are a significant cause of mortality in children (Lyen and Grant 1982; De Vile et al. 1996; Stripp et al. 2004).

Postoperative DI may be transient, permanent, or triphasic (Hollinshead 1964). In the majority of cases, AVP deficiency is transient, whereas prolonged polyuria occurs in no more than 10 % of patients (Hensen et al. 1999; Nemergut et al. 2005). The reason behind the large prevalence of transient vs. permanent DI is represented by the fact that about 90 % of AVP-secreting neurons need to degenerate in order to cause a permanent disease.

Transient DI usually arises within 1–2 days after surgery and disappears within a few days/1 week (Fig. 9.1). It is likely due to a temporary dysfunction of neurons that synthesize AVP; the dysfunction can be secondary to a traumatic disconnection between cell bodies and nerve terminals or to an axonal shock.

Triphasic DI is observed in about 3 % of patients undergoing transsphenoidal surgery. The first phase of triphasic DI appears to be originated by the same pathogenetic mechanisms of transient DI and is followed by a second phase of antidiuresis after about 1 week. This phase is characterized by an uncontrolled release of AVP, which is the hallmark of the syndrome of inappropriate antidiuresis (SIAD), from the degenerating nerve terminals (Hollinshead 1964). The shift from the first phase to the second phase of inappropriate antidiuresis is characterized by a decreased output of urine, which becomes concentrated. This sign should be carefully evaluated, because continued administration of an excess of fluids during this phase of antidiuresis can rapidly lead to hyponatremia. The second phase of triphasic DI can last from 2 to 14 days (Hensen et al. 1999; Nemergut et al. 2005). A minority of patients experience only the first two phases of triphasic DI. In patients with limited cell damage, only an isolated second phase may occur (Ultmann et al. 1992), which can be responsible for postsurgical hyponatremia in up to 20 % of patients (Hensen et al. 1999; Olson et al. 1995). The third phase of triphasic DI arises when AVP stores have been depleted and the majority of AVP-secreting neurons (about 90 %) have degenerated, thus leading to chronic DI.

In addition to SIAD, postsurgical hyponatremia may be caused by fluid overload during the perioperative period or, yet rarely, by the cerebral salt-wasting syndrome (CSWS) (Guerrero et al. 2007). In particular, the occurrence of CSWS after transsphenoidal surgery appears limited to the description of case reports (e.g., Andrews et al. 1986; Atkin et al. 1996; Filippella et al. 2002). CSWS is characterized by the

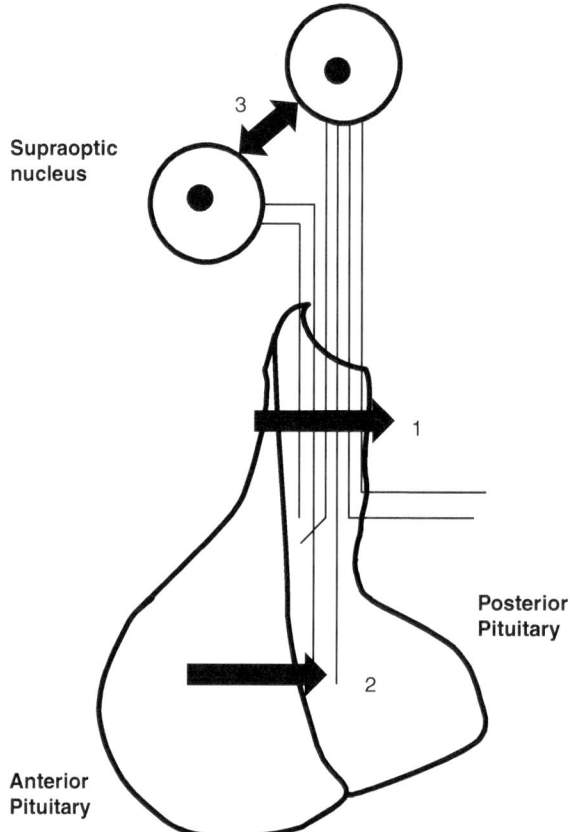

Fig. 9.1 Pathophysiology of postsurgical triphasic diabetes insipidus. (*1*) The first phase is caused by the section of the pituitary stalk (partial or complete) or by axonal shock. Consequently, the connection between the cell body of AVP-secreting neurons and nerve terminals in the posterior pituitary is interrupted, and this prevents AVP secretion. (*2*) The second phase is characterized by an uncontrolled release of AVP from degenerating nerve terminals. (*3*) The third phase may follow when the large majority (about 90 %) of AVP-secreting neurons in the hypothalamus (supraoptic and paraventricular nuclei) have degenerated

development of an excessive natriuresis occurring in patients with intracranial disease. Although the mechanisms underlying CSWS have not been completely elucidated, existing evidence involves the release of natriuretic factors [atrial natriuretic peptide (ANP), brain natriuretic peptide (BNP), C-type natriuretic peptide, and ouabain-like peptide]. This is accompanied by a decreased sympathetic input to the kidney. Together, these factors increase urinary sodium excretion and reduce effective arterial blood volume, which stimulates AVP release (Palmer 2003) (Fig. 9.2). The differential diagnosis between SIAD and CSWS may represent a difficult task, because the two conditions share some clinical and biochemical features. The

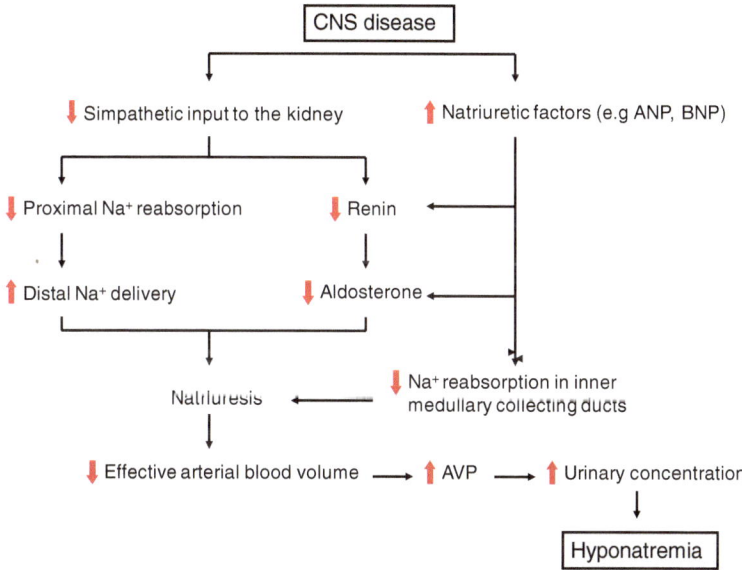

Fig. 9.2 Pathophysiology of CSWS. *ANP* atrial natriuretic peptide, *BNP* brain natriuretic peptide, *AVP* arginine vasopressin (Modified from Palmer 2003)

assessment of extracellular fluid volume is a key factor in the diagnostic workup, because CSWS is characterized by fluid volume depletion, whereas SIAD is substantially associated with a euvolemic status. It is crucial to differentiate these two conditions, because the treatment they require is different (Cole et al. 2004; Guerrero et al. 2007). It should be also kept in mind that late hyponatremia after transsphenoidal surgery may be caused by secondary adrenocortical insufficiency (Guerrero et al. 2007).

Recently, the case of a young patient (17-year-old), admitted for severe, yet asymptomatic, hypernatremia (173 mmol/l) and who had been diagnosed with CP at the age of 10 years and subjected to tumor resection and gamma knife surgery, has been reported (Kwon et al. 2012). Despite the high sodium level and the high serum osmolality (371 mOsm/kg H$_2$O), the patient did not report increased thirst. Based on laboratory assessment of the patient, which was indicative of hypertonic dehydration and acute non-oliguric renal failure due to dehydration, the authors suggested that hypernatremia had been induced by decreased thirst sensation secondary to CP and tumor resection. Thirst is normally stimulated by increased serum osmolality through cerebral osmoreceptors located in the vascular organ of the lamina terminalis. Organic lesions or surgical destruction of this anatomical structure may decrease the sensation of thirst in response to increased plasma osmolality. Admittedly, it appears reasonable to consider hypodipsic hypernatremia as a possible, yet likely rare, consequence of the presence of a brain lesion or of its resection.

9.4 Radiotherapy and Electrolyte Alterations

Radiotherapy in CP is used after limited surgery or in patients who are not candidates for surgery because the risks appear to outweigh the benefits. Irradiation can be performed with different modalities: conventional or conformal fractionated radiotherapy, intensity-modulated radiotherapy, proton beam radiotherapy, intracavitary application with yttrium-[90] or phosphorus-[32], or stereotactic radiotherapy, both in the form of stereotactic radiosurgery or fractionated stereotactic radiotherapy, which has been developed as a more accurate technique of irradiation with more precise tumor targeting (Fernandez-Miranda et al. 2011).

With regard to the effect of radiotherapy on posterior pituitary function, several reports on patients' outcomes after stereotactic radiotherapy indicate that the risk to develop DI as a direct consequence of this treatment appears to be very low. For example, in a series of 46 patients with CP subjected to stereotactic radiosurgery with gamma knife for residual or recurrent disease, no patient with normal pituitary function before radiotherapy developed hypopituitarism after 5 years of follow-up, including AVP deficiency (Niranjan et al. 2010). Similarly, in a pediatric series of patients, no case of DI was associated with the effects of radiotherapy after a follow-up of 6 years (Merchant et al. 2002). In another series of 98 patients with residual or recurrent CP and followed for over 5 years after gamma knife treatment, deterioration of endocrine function (not otherwise specified) was observed only in a very few cases (Kobayashi 2009). Overall, the published literature suggests that the onset of DI appears to be mainly a consequence of surgery rather than radiotherapy. This conclusion is in agreement with the results of a systematic review of studies publishing outcome data of a total of 540 patients treated for CP, which indicates that subtotal surgical removal followed by postoperative radiotherapy more likely preserves pituitary function, including normal AVP production, compared to gross total removal (Sughrue et al. 2011). These data confirm and reinforce similar conclusions of a previously published review on endocrine outcomes in patients treated for CP (Kalapurakal 2005). Nevertheless, long-term prospective studies are required to establish the potential of radiotherapy to minimize treatment-related adverse sequelae, including deterioration of endocrine functions.

9.5 Diagnosis

The possibility that a patient with CP develops DI should be considered when a patient excretes large volumes of diluted urine (in particular >2.5 ml/kg body weight/h), either before or after neurosurgery. In the latter case, patients typically present a sudden onset of polyuria and polydipsia, usually within 24–48 h after surgery (Loh and Verbalis 2007). Urine osmolality and specific gravity are reduced (<200 mOsm/kg H_2O and <1005, respectively). If present, serum hyperosmolality and hypernatremia are strong additional elements in support of a diagnosis of DI. However, because most patients maintain intact thirst mechanisms, they do not present increased serum osmolality or serum [Na⁺], as long as they have free access to oral fluids (Robertson 1995). This is the reason why it may be necessary to limit fluid intake and assess whether hyperosmolality and/or hypernatremia develop, in order to confirm a diagnosis of DI.

Besides DI, other etiologies leading to polyuria after surgery should be excluded. For instance, patients subjected to surgery in the suprasellar region often are treated with high doses of glucocorticoids in order to prevent the clinical manifestations associated with the possible presence of secondary adrenal failure (Loh and Verbalis 2007). Glucocorticoids may induce hyperglycemia and hence osmotic diuresis from glycosuria. In order to differentiate it from the polyuria induced by DI, urine and blood glucose should be measured. Another possible explanation for postsurgical polyuria may be the excess of fluids administered i.v. in the perioperative period, which may lead initially to hyponatremia. Serum [Na⁺] should be carefully monitored, in order to establish whether polyuria is the result of previous excessive fluid administration or is caused by DI. If hypotonic polyuria persists and is accompanied by the onset of hypernatremia and/or hyperosmolality, then the likely diagnosis is DI (Loh and Verbalis 2007). Imaging techniques may be helpful in the diagnostic workup, because the disappearance of the typical bright spot corresponding to the posterior pituitary on T_1-weighted images supports the diagnosis of DI (Tien et al. 1991). Nevertheless, it should be considered that the bright spot may still be seen at early phases of DI, and therefore its presence cannot exclude the presence of the disease (Maghnie et al. 1997).

As mentioned previously, postoperative hyponatremia may occur due to different conditions, but it is mainly secondary to SIAD. The essential diagnostic criteria of SIAD are shown in Table 9.1 (Ellison and Berl 2007). SIAD may have to be distinguished from CSWS, as already mentioned, although the latter rarely occurs after surgery for CP. Some features of CSWS are virtually identical to those observed in SIAD, namely, hypotonic hyponatremia without maximally diluted urine and urinary sodium retention. However, at variance with SIAD, which is substantially characterized by a euvolemic status, CSWS is characterized by a hypovolemic status, as mentioned previously. Some laboratory indexes, which may be helpful in differentiating the two conditions, are reported in Table 9.2 (Cole et al. 2004).

Table 9.1 Essential diagnostic criteria of SIAD	Essential features of SIAD
	Decreased serum osmolality (<275 mOsm/kg H₂O)
	Urinary osmolality >100 mOsm/kg H₂O during hypotonicity
	Clinical euvolemia
	No clinical signs of contraction or expansion of extracellular fluid
	Urinary sodium >40 mmol/l with normal dietary salt intake
	Normal thyroid and adrenal function
	No recent use of diuretic agents
	Modified from Ellison and Berl (2007)

Table 9.2 Laboratory
parameters that may be useful
for the differential diagnosis
between CSWS and SIAD

	CSWS	SIAD
Extracellular volume	↓	=
Hematocrit	↑	=/↓
Serum albumin	↑	=
BUN	↑	=/↓
Serum creatinine	↑	=/↓

BUN= blood urea nitrogen

9.6   Treatment

Patients with DI at the time of the diagnosis of CP or diagnosed following surgery or radiotherapy will benefit from desmopressin treatment, which effectively reduces urine output. A dose of 1–2 mcg (i.v. or s.c) can be administered initially. It is of pivotal importance to monitor urine volume and osmolality and serum [Na$^+$] at regular intervals, in order to determine the appropriate dose and frequency of administration. In practice, the excretion of 200–250 ml/h of diluted urine (osmolality <200 mOsm/kg H$_2$O) suggests the need for a repeated dose of desmopressin (Verbalis 2003).

Patients with postsurgical DI deserve particular attention, because this condition may be transient, permanent, or triphasic, as previously said. The transition from a polyuric phase to serum hypo-osmolality may suggest a shift to SIAD (in triphasic diabetes insipidus) and should be carefully monitored, in order to promptly stop desmopressin administration, possibly before the onset of hyponatremia. Nevertheless, hyponatremia may occur, and it has to be considered that it may be also secondary to an excessive dose of desmopressin, besides SIAD. The discontinuation of desmopressin followed by frequent serum [Na$^+$] measurements (i.e., every 6–8 h) should clarify whether the patient is experiencing or not a phase of antidiuresis. A positive daily fluid balance >2 l supports the transition to a phase of inappropriate antidiuresis. Desmopressin has a short half-life (≤20 min), and therefore its effect can be rapidly terminated upon treatment discontinuation. On the other hand, failure to stop desmopressin administration can lead to cerebral edema and possibly to dramatic consequences (Bohn et al. 2005).

It is also important to monitor fluid replacement in patients with postoperative DI. Whenever possible, the patient should be allowed to drink in response to thirst, which is normally stimulated by a 2–3 % increase of serum osmolality (Robertson 1983). In case the patient is unable to drink, fluids should be administered i.v. The following formula can be of help in estimating water deficit: $0.6 \times$ (serum [Na$^+$/140] − 1). If a phase of inappropriate antidiuresis occurs, fluids should be restricted in order to maintain serum [Na$^+$] within the normal range. Conversely, in those rare cases in which clinical and biochemical features are indicative of the presence of CSWS, isotonic fluids should be administered.

It should be also reminded the possible presence of anterior pituitary hormone deficiencies, in particular of ACTH, because secondary adrenocortical insufficiency may lead to hyponatremia, which can be counteracted by corticosteroids supplementation. In clinical practice, because any patient with postoperative DI may also have anterior pituitary insufficiency, hydrocortisone (50–100 mg i.v. every 8 h) is usually administered immediately after surgery, and it is subsequently tapered to a dose of 15–25 mg per day until anterior pituitary function can be assessed (Loh and Verbalis 2007).

In patients with chronic DI desmopressin treatment will be prolonged indefinitely, usually with oral or intranasal administration of the drug. The oral route requires doses (200–400 μg 2–4 times per day) that are about 20 times higher than the intranasal route, because the large majority of oral desmopressin (>99 %) is destroyed by gastrointestinal peptidases.

Conclusions

Water-electrolyte imbalance may be present in CP both at the time of diagnosis and after treatment, particularly after surgical procedures. Patients should be carefully monitored, especially in the perioperative period, and in case water-electrolyte alterations occur, the possible etiology should be thoroughly investigated in order to warrant the most effective intervention. Particular attention deserves the possible occurrence of the triphasic DI, which admittedly challenges the ability of the clinician to appropriately manage this type of alteration.

References

Ahmed S, Elsheikh M, Stratton IM et al (1999) Outcome of transsphenoidal surgery for acromegaly and its relationship to surgical experience. Clin Endocrinol 50:561–567

Andrews BT, Fitzgerald PA, Tyrell JB et al (1986) Cerebral salt wasting after pituitary exploration and biopsy: case report. Neurosurgery 18:469–471

Atkin SL, Coady AM, White MC et al (1996) Hyponatraemia secondary to cerebral salt wasting syndrome following routine pituitary surgery. Eur J Endocrinol 135:245–247

Bohn D, Davids MR, Friedman O et al (2005) Acute and fatal hyponatraemia after resection of a craniopharyngioma: a preventable tragedy. QJM 98:691–703

Campbell PG, McGettigan B, Luginbuhl A et al (2010) Endocrinological and ophthalmological consequences of an initial endonasal endoscopic approach for resection of craniopharyngiomas. Neurosurg Focus 28:E8

Cavallo LM, Prevedello DM, Solari D et al (2009) Extended endoscopic endonasal transsphenoidal approach for residual or recurrent craniopharyngiomas. J Neurosurg 111:578–589

Cole CD, Gottfried ON, Liu JK et al (2004) Hyponatremia in the neurosurgical patient: diagnosis and management. Neurosurg Focus 16:1–10

De Vile CJ, Grant DB, Hayward RD et al (1996) Growth and endocrine sequelae of craniopharyngioma. Arch Dis Child 75:108–114

Ellison DH, Berl T (2007) The syndrome of inappropriate antidiuresis. N Engl J Med 356:2064–2072

Fahlbusch R, Honegger J, Paulus W et al (1999) Surgical treatment of craniopharyngiomas: experience with 168 patients. J Neurosurg 90:237–250

Fatemi N, Dusick JR, de Paiva Neto MA et al (2009) Endonasal versus supraorbital keyhole removal of craniopharyngiomas and tuberculum sellae meningiomas. Neurosurgery 64(Suppl 2):269–284

Fernandez-Miranda JC, Gardner PA, Snyderman CH et al (2011) Craniopharyngioma: a patho-logic, clinical, and surgical review. Head Neck 34:1036–1044

Filippella M, Cappabianca P, Cavallo LM et al (2002) Very delayed hyponatremia after surgery and radiotherapy for a pituitary macroadenoma. J Endocrinol Invest 25:163–168

Gardner PA, Kassam AB, Snyderman CH et al (2008) Outcomes following endoscopic, expanded endonasal resection of suprasellar craniopharyngiomas: a case series. J Neurosurg 109:6–16

Guerrero R, Pumar A, Soto A, Pomares MA et al (2007) Early hyponatraemia after pituitary sur-gery: cerebral salt-wasting syndrome. Eur J Endocrinol 156:611–616

Hensen J, Henig A, Fahlbusch R et al (1999) Prevalence, predictors and patterns of postoperative polyuria and hyponatraemia in the immediate course after transsphenoidal surgery for pituitary adenomas. Clin Endocrinol 50:431–439

Hetelekidis S, Barnes PD, Tao ML et al (1993) 20-year experience in childhood craniopharyngi-oma. Int J Radiat Oncol Biol Phys 27:189–195

Hollinshead WH (1964) The interphase of diabetes insipidus. Mayo Clin Proc 39:92–100

Honegger J, Buchfelder M, Fahlbusch R (1999) Surgical treatment of craniopharyngiomas: endo-crinological results. J Neurosurg 90:251–257

Jane JA Jr, Kiehna E, Payne SC et al (2010) Early outcomes of endoscopic transsphenoidal surgery for adult craniopharyngiomas. Neurosurg Focus 28, E9

Kalapurakal JA (2005) Radiation therapy in the management of pediatric craniopharyngiomas--a review. Childs Nerv Syst 21:808–816

Karavitaki N, Brufani C, Warner JT et al (2005) Craniopharyngiomas in children and adults: sys-tematic analysis of 121 cases with long-term follow-up. Clin Endocrinol 62:397–409

Karavitaki N, Cudlip S, Adams CB et al (2006) Craniopharyngiomas. Endocr Rev 27:371–397

Karavitaki N, Wass JAH (2008) Craniopharyngiomas. Endocrinol Metab Clin North Am 37:173–193

Kobayashi T (2009) Long-term results of gamma knife radiosurgery for 100 consecutive cases of craniopharyngioma and a treatment strategy. Prog Neurol Surg 22:63–76

Kwon AR, Ann JM, Shin JI et al (2012) Hypodipsic hypernatremia leading to reversible renal failure following surgery for craniopharyngioma. J Pediatr Endocrinol Metab 25:1027–1030

Leroy C, Karrouz W, Douillard C et al (2013) Diabetes insipidus. Ann Endocrinol (Paris) 74:496–507

Loh JA, Verbalis JG (2007) Diabetes insipidus as a complication after pituitary surgery. Nat Clin Pract Endocrinol Metab 3:489–494

Lyen KR, Grant DB (1982) Endocrine function, morbidity, and mortality after surgery for cranio-pharyngioma. Arch Dis Child 57:837–841

Maghnie M, Genovese E, Bernasconi S et al (1997) Persistent high MR signal of the posterior pituitary gland in central diabetes insipidus. AJNR Am J Neuroradiol 18:1749–1752

Merchant TE, Kiehna EN, Sanford RA et al (2002) Craniopharyngioma: the St. Jude Children's Research Hospital experience 1984–2001. Int J Radiat Oncol Biol Phys 53:533–542

Müller HL, Kaatsch P, Warmuth-Metz M et al (2003) Childhood craniopharyngioma-diagnostic and therapeutic strategies. Monatsschr Kinderheilkd 151:1056–1063

Müller HL (2010) Childhood craniopharyngioma–current concepts in diagnosis, therapy and fol-low-up. Nat Rev Endocrinol 6:609–618

Murad MH, Fernández-Balsells MM, Barwise A et al (2010) Outcomes of surgical treatment for nonfunctioning pituitary adenomas: a systematic review and meta-analysis. Clin Endocrinol 73:777–791

Nemergut EC, Zuo Z, Jane JA Jr et al (2005) Predictors of diabetes insipidus after transsphenoidal surgery: a review of 881 patients. J Neurosurg 103:448–454

Niranjan A, Kano H, Mathieu D et al (2010) Radiosurgery for craniopharyngioma. Int J Radiat Oncol Biol Phys 78:64–71

Olson BR, Rubino D, Gumowski J et al (1995) Isolated hyponatremia after transsphenoidal pitu-itary surgery. J Clin Endocrinol Metab 80:85–91

Paja M, Lucas T, Garcia-Uria F et al (1995) Hypothalamic-pituitary dysfunction in patients with craniopharyngioma. Clin Endocrinol 42:467–473

Palmer BF (2003) Hyponatremia in patient with central nervous system disease: SIADH versus CSW. Trends Endocrinol Metab 14:182–187

Pratheesh R, Swallow DMA, Rajaratnam S et al (2013) Incidence, predictors and early postoperative course of diabetes insipidus in paediatric craniopharyngioma: a comparison with adults. Childs Nerv Syst 29:941–949

Robertson GL (1983) Thirst and vasopressin function in normal and disordered states of water balance. J Lab Clin Med 101:351–371

Robertson GL (1995) Diabetes insipidus. Endocrinol Metab Clin North Am 24:549–557

Stripp DC, Maity A, Janss AJ et al (2004) Surgery with or without radiation therapy in the management of craniopharyngiomas in children and young adults. Int J Radiat Oncol Biol Phys 58:714–720

Sughrue ME, Yang I, Kane AJ et al (2011) Endocrinologic, neurologic, and visual morbidity after treatment for craniopharyngioma. J Neurooncol 101:463–476

Thomsett MJ, Conte FA, Kaplan SL (1980) Endocrine and neurologic outcome in childhood craniopharyngioma: review of effect of treatment in 42 patients. J Pediatr 97:728–735

Tien R, Kucharczyk J, Kucharczyk W (1991) MR imaging of the brain in patients with diabetes insipidus. Am J Neuroradiol 12:533–542

Ultmann MC, Hoffman GE, Nelson PB et al (1992) Transient hyponatremia after damage to the neurohypophyseal tracts. Neuroendocrinol 56:803–811

Van Effenterre R, Boch AL (2002) Craniopharyngioma in adults and children: a study of 122 surgical cases. J Neurosurg 97:3–11

Verbalis JG (2003) Diabetes insipidus. Rev Endocr Metab Disord 4:177–185